The Essential Exocrine Pancreatic Insufficiency (EPI) Cookbook for New Diagnoses 2024

Comprehensive Guide to EPI, Expert Guidance, Essential Recipes, and Lifestyle Hacks for Thriving with Exocrine Pancreatic Insufficiency

Dr. Sarah Matthews

Copyright © 2024 by Dr. Sarah Matthews

All rights reserved.

No part of this book may be reproduced, distributed, or transmitted in any form or by any means, including photocopying, recording, or other electronic or mechanical methods, without the prior written permission of the publisher, except in the case of brief quotations embodied in critical reviews and certain other noncommercial uses permitted by copyright law.

TABLE OF CONTENTS

Foreword
- Acknowledgments
- About the Author

Introduction
- Understanding Exocrine Pancreatic Insufficiency (EPI)
- Overview of the Book

Chapter 1: Demystifying EPI
- What is Exocrine Pancreatic Insufficiency?
- Causes and Risk Factors
- Symptoms and Diagnosis

Chapter 2: Getting Started with EPI
- Coping with the Diagnosis
- Building Your Support Network
- Communicating with Healthcare Providers

Chapter 3: The EPI Diet: Foundation for Wellness
- Principles of the EPI Diet
- Essential Nutrients for EPI Management
- Tailoring Your Diet to Your Needs

Chapter 4: Navigating Nutrition with EPI
- Understanding Enzyme Replacement Therapy (ERT)

- Optimizing Enzyme Use with Meals and Snacks
- Exploring Dietary Supplements

Chapter 5: The EPI Cookbook: Essential Recipes and Meal Plans

- Breakfasts for Digestive Ease
- Lunches to Fuel Your Day
- Dinners for Digestive Delight
- Snacks and Treats for Every Craving
- Sample Meal Plans for Different Dietary Preferences

Chapter 6: Lifestyle Strategies for EPI Management

- Managing Digestive Symptoms
- Balancing Physical Activity and Rest
- Coping with Emotional Challenges

Chapter 7: Beyond the Plate: Holistic Approaches to EPI

- Mindfulness and Stress Reduction Techniques
- Integrative Therapies for Digestive Support
- Advocating for Yourself and Others

Chapter 8: Living Your Best Life with EPI

- Setting Goals and Celebrating Successes
- Traveling and Dining Out with Confidence
- Inspiring Stories of Individuals Thriving with EPI

Conclusion

- Looking Ahead: Advances in EPI Research and Treatment
- Final Thoughts

Appendices

- Glossary of Terms
- Resources for Further Reading
- Index

Foreword

Welcome to "The Essential Exocrine Pancreatic Insufficiency (EPI) Cookbook for New Diagnoses 2024." In the pages of this cookbook, you'll embark on a transformative journey of culinary exploration and empowerment. As someone newly diagnosed with Exocrine Pancreatic Insufficiency (EPI), you may be navigating uncharted waters, facing questions, concerns, and perhaps even a bit of uncertainty about how to manage this condition. Fear not, for within these recipes and insights lies the power to reclaim control over your health and well-being.

Acknowledgments

Before we dive into the flavorful world of EPI-friendly cuisine, I extend my deepest gratitude to the individuals and institutions whose contributions have made this cookbook possible. To the healthcare professionals and researchers tirelessly dedicated to advancing our understanding and treatment of EPI, your expertise and compassion are the cornerstone of hope for those affected by this condition. To the courageous individuals living with EPI who generously shared their experiences, challenges, and triumphs, your resilience and strength inspire us all. And to my own support network of family, friends, and colleagues, thank you for your unwavering encouragement and belief in the transformative power of food.

About the Author

Allow me to introduce myself. I am Dr. Sarah Matthews, a passionate advocate for health and wellness with a specialization in gastroenterology and nutrition. As a board-certified gastroenterologist with over a decade of experience, I have dedicated my career to helping individuals navigate digestive health challenges, including Exocrine Pancreatic Insufficiency (EPI). My expertise extends beyond the clinic to the kitchen, where I believe that food can be a powerful tool for healing and nourishment. With a deep understanding of the physiological mechanisms underlying EPI and a flair for creating delicious, EPI-friendly recipes, I am thrilled to share my knowledge and passion with you in this cookbook. Together, let's unlock the power of nutrition and embark on a journey to thrive with EPI.

INTRODUCTION

Greetings, fellow culinary enthusiasts! I am Dr. Sarah Matthews, and for more than two decades, I've embarked on a mission to empower individuals navigating the labyrinth of Exocrine Pancreatic Insufficiency (EPI). Picture this: a bustling kitchen filled with the tantalizing aromas of spices and herbs, where every sizzle, chop, and stir tells a story of resilience and triumph over adversity.

EPI is not just a medical diagnosis; it's a journey filled with twists, turns, and unexpected detours. Imagine standing at the crossroads of health, uncertainty casting its shadow over every decision, every meal. It's a challenge I've witnessed firsthand in the eyes of patients like Emma, whose journey from diagnosis to empowerment inspired the creation of this cookbook.

Emma's story resonates deeply, reminding us of the diverse experiences that thread through these pages. Within these culinary corridors, you'll find more than just recipes; you'll discover a roadmap to reclaiming your relationship with food and embracing the art of nourishment.

Join me on this gastronomic odyssey as we unlock the secrets of nutrition, one delectable dish at a time. Together, let's turn fear into flavor, uncertainty into exploration, and isolation into community. For in the kitchen, where ingredients dance and flavors sing, we find not just sustenance, but solace, connection, and the boundless potential for healing.

Welcome to "The Essential Exocrine Pancreatic Insufficiency (EPI) Cookbook for New Diagnoses 2024." Let the culinary adventure begin!

Understanding Exocrine Pancreatic Insufficiency (EPI)

Exocrine Pancreatic Insufficiency (EPI) is a complex condition that impacts the digestive system, specifically the pancreas. This crucial organ, nestled behind the stomach, plays a vital role in the digestion and absorption of nutrients. However, when EPI strikes, the pancreas becomes compromised, hindering its ability to produce and release essential digestive enzymes.

These enzymes—lipase, protease, and amylase—are like culinary alchemists, breaking down fats, proteins, and carbohydrates into smaller molecules that the body can absorb and utilize. Without an adequate supply of these enzymes, the process of digestion falters, leading to a cascade of symptoms and complications.

Imagine a well-oiled machine suddenly sputtering and stalling, unable to perform its essential functions. That's the reality faced by individuals with EPI. Symptoms may vary from person to person but often include abdominal discomfort, bloating, gas, diarrhea, weight loss, and malnutrition.

Diagnosing EPI can be challenging, as its symptoms overlap with those of other gastrointestinal disorders. However, healthcare providers employ a variety of diagnostic tests, including blood tests, stool tests, imaging studies, and pancreatic function tests, to confirm a diagnosis.

Understanding EPI is the first step towards managing and overcoming its challenges. By unraveling the complexities of this condition, we empower ourselves to make informed decisions about our health and well-being.

Throughout this cookbook, we'll delve deeper into the causes, symptoms, diagnosis, and management strategies for EPI, providing you with the knowledge and tools to navigate this journey with confidence.

Overview of the Book

"EPI Essentials 2024: The Ultimate Cookbook for New Diagnoses" is more than just a collection of recipes; it's a comprehensive guide designed to support individuals newly diagnosed with Exocrine Pancreatic Insufficiency (EPI) on their journey to better health and well-being. Within the pages of this cookbook, you'll find a treasure trove of knowledge, inspiration, and practical tools to navigate the challenges of EPI with confidence and creativity.

- **Expert Guidance**

From understanding the fundamentals of EPI to learning about the latest advancements in treatment and management, this book offers expert guidance from healthcare professionals specializing in gastroenterology, nutrition, and culinary arts. You'll gain insights into the underlying mechanisms of EPI, its impact on digestion and nutrition, and strategies for optimizing your dietary choices to support digestive health.

- **Essential Recipes**

Discover a diverse array of mouthwatering recipes crafted specifically with the needs of individuals with EPI in mind. From hearty breakfasts to satisfying dinners, each recipe is carefully designed to be delicious, nutritious, and easy to digest. Whether you're craving comforting classics or exploring new culinary frontiers, you'll find something to tantalize your taste buds in this cookbook.

- **Practical Meal Plans**

Take the guesswork out of meal planning with practical and customizable meal plans tailored to your dietary preferences and nutritional needs. Whether you're following a low-fat diet, gluten-free regimen, or vegetarian lifestyle, these meal plans provide a roadmap to delicious and balanced eating, ensuring that you never feel deprived or overwhelmed by your dietary restrictions.

- **Lifestyle Hacks**

Beyond the kitchen, this book offers lifestyle hacks and tips for thriving with EPI in every aspect of life. From managing symptoms and navigating social situations to traveling and dining out with confidence, you'll discover practical strategies for living your best life with EPI.

- **Empowerment**

Above all, "EPI Essentials 2024" is about empowerment. It's about equipping you with the knowledge, skills, and confidence to take control of your health and well-being. Whether you're newly diagnosed with EPI or have been living with the condition for years, this cookbook is your companion on the journey to a healthier, happier you.

CHAPTER 1

DEMYSTIFYING EPI

Exocrine Pancreatic Insufficiency (EPI) is a gastrointestinal disorder characterized by the inadequate production or secretion of digestive enzymes by the pancreas. These enzymes are essential for breaking down fats, proteins, and carbohydrates in the food we consume. Without enough enzymes, the digestive process is compromised, leading to malabsorption and a range of symptoms.

EPI can arise from various underlying conditions or factors that impair the function of the pancreas. Chronic pancreatitis, cystic fibrosis, pancreatic cancer, and pancreatic surgery are among the primary causes of EPI. Lifestyle factors such as excessive alcohol consumption and smoking can also contribute to its development.

The symptoms of EPI can vary but commonly include abdominal pain, bloating, gas, diarrhea, weight loss, and nutrient deficiencies. Diagnosis is typically made through a combination of medical history, physical examination, blood tests, stool tests, imaging studies, and pancreatic function tests.

Understanding EPI is crucial for effective management and treatment. Early detection and diagnosis enable healthcare providers to initiate appropriate interventions, improve symptom control, and prevent complications associated with EPI.

What is Exocrine Pancreatic Insufficiency?

Exocrine Pancreatic Insufficiency (EPI) is a gastrointestinal disorder characterized by the insufficient production or secretion of digestive enzymes by the pancreas. To comprehend EPI fully, it's crucial to delve into the intricate anatomy and function of this vital organ.

Anatomy and Function of the Pancreas:

The pancreas, nestled behind the stomach in the upper abdomen, serves both endocrine and exocrine functions. In its exocrine role, it produces and releases digestive enzymes—lipase, protease, and amylase—into the small intestine to aid in food digestion.

When food enters the small intestine, the pancreas secretes these enzymes in response to hormonal signals. These enzymes then act like molecular scissors, cutting large molecules of fats, proteins, and carbohydrates into smaller fragments that can be easily absorbed by the intestine.

Impact of Insufficient Enzyme Production:

In individuals with EPI, the pancreas fails to produce an adequate amount of these digestive enzymes, leading to impaired digestion and nutrient absorption. Without sufficient enzymes, fats, proteins, and carbohydrates remain undigested, resulting in malabsorption and a range of gastrointestinal symptoms.

Causes of Exocrine Pancreatic Insufficiency:

EPI can arise from various underlying conditions or factors that impair pancreatic function. Chronic pancreatitis, cystic fibrosis, pancreatic cancer, pancreatic surgery, and autoimmune conditions affecting the pancreas are primary causes of EPI. Lifestyle factors such as excessive alcohol consumption and smoking can also contribute to its development.

Symptoms of Exocrine Pancreatic Insufficiency:

The symptoms of EPI can vary but commonly include abdominal pain, bloating, gas, diarrhea, weight loss, and nutrient deficiencies. These symptoms arise due to impaired digestion and malabsorption of fats, proteins, and carbohydrates.

Diagnostic Process:

Diagnosing EPI involves a multifaceted approach, beginning with a thorough medical history and physical examination. Healthcare providers may order blood tests to measure enzyme levels, stool tests to assess fat content, and imaging studies (such as CT scans or MRI) to evaluate pancreatic function. Additionally, pancreatic function tests may be performed to confirm the diagnosis.

Treatment and Management:

Treatment for EPI typically revolves around enzyme replacement therapy, which involves taking synthetic digestive enzymes with meals to aid in digestion. Additionally, dietary modifications, nutritional supplements, and lifestyle changes may be recommended to manage symptoms and optimize digestive health.

Understanding the complex interplay between pancreatic anatomy, enzyme function, and the development of Exocrine Pancreatic Insufficiency is essential for effective diagnosis, treatment, and management of the condition.

Causes and Risk Factors

Exocrine Pancreatic Insufficiency (EPI) can arise from various underlying conditions or factors that impair the function of the pancreas. Understanding these causes and risk factors is essential for identifying individuals at risk and implementing appropriate preventive measures and treatments.

Primary Causes:

1. **Chronic Pancreatitis:** Long-term inflammation of the pancreas can lead to damage and scarring of pancreatic tissue, impairing its ability to produce and release digestive enzymes.

2. **Cystic Fibrosis:** This genetic disorder affects the production of mucus, sweat, and digestive fluids, including pancreatic enzymes.

Individuals with cystic fibrosis often experience EPI due to the blockage of pancreatic ducts by thickened mucus.

3. **Pancreatic Cancer:** Tumors in the pancreas can obstruct the flow of digestive enzymes, leading to EPI. Additionally, treatments such as surgery or radiation therapy may damage pancreatic tissue, further exacerbating the condition.

4. **Pancreatic Surgery:** Surgical procedures involving the pancreas, such as pancreaticoduodenectomy (Whipple procedure), can disrupt normal pancreatic function and contribute to the development of EPI.

5. **Autoimmune Conditions:** Autoimmune diseases affecting the pancreas, such as autoimmune pancreatitis, can result in inflammation and damage to pancreatic tissue, leading to EPI.

Secondary Factors:

1. **Alcohol Consumption:** Excessive alcohol consumption over a prolonged period can cause inflammation of the pancreas (pancreatitis), increasing the risk of EPI.

2. **Smoking:** Smoking is associated with an increased risk of developing chronic pancreatitis, a common precursor to EPI.

Other Risk Factors:

- **Family History:** Individuals with a family history of pancreatic diseases or EPI may have a higher risk of developing the condition.

- **Age:** EPI can occur at any age but is more commonly diagnosed in adults, particularly those over the age of 40.

- **Genetic Factors:** Certain genetic mutations and predispositions may increase the likelihood of developing EPI, particularly in individuals with a family history of the condition.

By identifying and addressing these underlying causes and risk factors, healthcare providers can take proactive measures to prevent, diagnose, and manage Exocrine Pancreatic Insufficiency effectively.

Symptoms and Diagnosis

Exocrine Pancreatic Insufficiency (EPI) presents with a variety of symptoms that can vary in severity and impact on an individual's quality of life. Recognizing these symptoms and undergoing proper diagnostic evaluation are essential steps in effectively managing the condition.

Common Symptoms of EPI:

1. **Abdominal Pain:** Individuals with EPI may experience persistent or recurrent abdominal pain, which can vary in intensity and location.

2. **Bloating and Gas:** Excessive gas production and bloating are common symptoms of EPI, often accompanied by abdominal discomfort.

3. **Diarrhea:** Diarrhea is a frequent symptom of EPI, characterized by loose, watery stools that may be foul-smelling and difficult to control.

4. **Weight Loss:** Malabsorption of nutrients due to inadequate digestion can lead to unintentional weight loss in individuals with EPI.

5. **Nutrient Deficiencies:** Insufficient absorption of fats, proteins, and carbohydrates can result in nutrient deficiencies, leading to fatigue, weakness, and other health complications.

Diagnostic Process:

Diagnosing EPI involves a comprehensive evaluation by a healthcare provider, including a thorough medical history, physical examination, and diagnostic tests. Key steps in the diagnostic process include:

1. **Medical History:** Healthcare providers will inquire about symptoms, medical history, family history, and lifestyle factors that may contribute to the development of EPI.

2. **Physical Examination:** A physical examination may reveal signs such as abdominal tenderness, distension, or signs of malnutrition.

3. **Blood Tests:** Blood tests may be performed to measure levels of pancreatic enzymes, such as amylase and lipase, as well as markers of malabsorption, such as vitamin and mineral levels.

4. **Stool Tests:** Stool tests may be used to assess fat content and the presence of undigested food particles, indicating malabsorption.

5. **Imaging Studies:** Imaging studies, such as abdominal ultrasound, CT scan, or MRI, may be ordered to evaluate the structure and function of the pancreas and surrounding organs.

6. **Pancreatic Function Tests:** Specialized tests, such as the secretin stimulation test or the fecal elastase test, may be performed to assess pancreatic function and confirm the diagnosis of EPI.

Importance of Early Diagnosis:

Early diagnosis of EPI is crucial for initiating appropriate treatment and preventing complications associated with malnutrition and nutrient deficiencies. By recognizing the symptoms and undergoing timely diagnostic evaluation, individuals with EPI can receive prompt intervention and support to improve their quality of life.

CHAPTER 2

GETTING STARTED WITH EPI

Exocrine Pancreatic Insufficiency (EPI) can be overwhelming, especially for individuals newly diagnosed with the condition. This chapter serves as a guide to help you navigate the initial stages of managing EPI, from understanding your diagnosis to making lifestyle adjustments and accessing resources for support.

Understanding Your Diagnosis:

Upon receiving a diagnosis of EPI, it's natural to have questions and concerns about what it means for your health and well-being. Take the time to discuss your diagnosis with your healthcare provider, ask questions, and seek clarification on any aspects you may not fully understand. Understanding the nature of EPI and its impact on your digestive health is the first step toward effectively managing the condition.

Educating Yourself About EPI:

Knowledge is empowering when it comes to managing EPI. Take advantage of reputable sources of information, such as medical websites, books, and support groups, to learn more about the condition, its causes, symptoms, treatment options, and lifestyle modifications. Educating yourself about EPI will enable you to make informed decisions about your health and actively participate in your treatment plan.

Creating a Support Network:

Living with EPI can be challenging, but you don't have to navigate it alone. Reach out to friends, family members, and peers who can offer understanding, encouragement, and support. Consider joining online forums or support groups for individuals with EPI to connect with others who share similar experiences and gain valuable insights and advice.

Making Dietary Adjustments:

Diet plays a crucial role in managing EPI and optimizing digestive health. Work with a registered dietitian or nutritionist to develop a personalized meal plan tailored to your specific needs and dietary preferences. Focus on consuming foods that are easily digestible and nutrient-rich, while minimizing foods that may exacerbate symptoms or trigger digestive discomfort.

Exploring Treatment Options:

Treatment for EPI typically involves enzyme replacement therapy, which involves taking synthetic digestive enzymes with meals to aid in digestion. Your healthcare provider may also recommend other medications, nutritional supplements, or interventions to manage symptoms and improve your overall quality of life. Discuss your treatment options with your healthcare team to determine the most suitable approach for you.

Planning for the Future:

Living with EPI is a journey, and it's essential to approach it with a long-term perspective. Take proactive steps to manage your condition, prioritize your health and well-being, and plan for the future. Stay engaged with your healthcare team, attend regular check-ups, and monitor your symptoms closely to ensure timely intervention and optimal management of EPI.

Coping with the Diagnosis

Receiving a diagnosis of Exocrine Pancreatic Insufficiency (EPI) can evoke a range of emotions, from shock and disbelief to fear and uncertainty. Coping with the diagnosis involves navigating these emotions, adjusting to the realities of living with a chronic condition, and finding strategies to maintain your physical and emotional well-being.

Acknowledge Your Feelings:

It's normal to experience a whirlwind of emotions upon receiving a diagnosis of EPI. Allow yourself to acknowledge and express your feelings, whether it's sadness, anger, frustration, or anxiety. Talking to a trusted friend, family member, or mental health professional can provide a safe space to process your emotions and gain perspective on your situation.

Seek Information and Support:

Knowledge is empowering when it comes to coping with EPI. Educate yourself about the condition, its causes, symptoms, treatment options, and lifestyle adjustments. Take advantage of reputable sources of information, such as medical websites, books, and support groups, to gain insights and connect with others who understand what you're going through.

Focus on What You Can Control:

While living with EPI may present challenges, focus on what you can control rather than dwelling on what you can't. Take proactive steps to manage your condition, such as adhering to your treatment plan, making dietary adjustments, practicing good self-care, and seeking support when needed. By taking ownership of your health and well-being, you can enhance your sense of control and resilience.

Build a Support Network:

Surround yourself with a supportive network of friends, family members, and healthcare professionals who can offer understanding, encouragement, and practical assistance. Don't hesitate to reach out for help when you need it, whether it's for emotional support, assistance with daily tasks, or navigating healthcare challenges. Building a strong support network can provide a valuable source of strength and comfort as you cope with the challenges of living with EPI.

Practice Self-Care:

Taking care of your physical and emotional well-being is essential when living with a chronic condition like EPI. Incorporate self-care practices into your daily routine, such as regular exercise, healthy eating, adequate sleep, stress management techniques, and activities that bring you joy and relaxation. Prioritizing self-care can help you maintain your overall health and resilience in the face of adversity.

Stay Positive and Hopeful:

Maintaining a positive outlook and cultivating a sense of hope can be powerful tools for coping with EPI. Focus on the things that bring you joy and fulfillment, set realistic goals for yourself, and celebrate your achievements, no matter how small. Remember that living with EPI is a journey, and there will be ups and downs along the way. Stay optimistic and resilient, and remember that you're not alone in facing this challenge.

Building Your Support Network

Living with Exocrine Pancreatic Insufficiency (EPI) can be challenging, but you don't have to navigate it alone. Building a support network of friends, family members, healthcare professionals, and peers who understand your journey can provide invaluable support, encouragement, and practical assistance along the way.

Identifying Supportive Individuals:

Start by identifying individuals in your life who are supportive, understanding, and willing to offer assistance when needed. This may include family members, close friends, coworkers, neighbors, and members of your community who can provide emotional support, companionship, and practical help with daily tasks.

Seeking Support from Healthcare Professionals:

Your healthcare team, including your primary care physician, gastroenterologist, dietitian, and mental health professional, plays a crucial role in supporting you in managing EPI. Don't hesitate to reach out to your healthcare providers for guidance, advice, and treatment options tailored to your needs. They can offer medical expertise, monitor your condition, and adjust your treatment plan as needed to optimize your health and well-being.

Connecting with Peers:

Connecting with others who are living with EPI can provide a unique source of understanding, empathy, and shared experiences. Consider joining online forums, support groups, or local community organizations for individuals with EPI or digestive health conditions. These platforms offer opportunities to share insights, exchange advice, and gain support from others who are facing similar challenges.

Educating Your Support Network:

It's essential to educate your support network about EPI, its symptoms, treatment options, and lifestyle adjustments. Help them understand your condition, its impact on your daily life, and the ways in which they can offer support and assistance. Open and honest communication fosters understanding, empathy, and effective collaboration in managing EPI together.

Expressing Your Needs:

Be proactive in expressing your needs, preferences, and concerns to your support network. Whether you require emotional support, assistance with daily tasks, or someone to accompany you to medical appointments, don't hesitate to communicate your needs clearly and assertively. Your support network is there to help you, but they may not always know how best to support you unless you communicate your needs openly.

Showing Appreciation:

Take the time to show appreciation for the support and assistance you receive from your network. Express gratitude for their presence, understanding, and willingness to help, whether through a heartfelt thank-you note, a thoughtful gesture, or simply acknowledging their support verbally. Showing appreciation strengthens your relationships and reinforces the bonds of your support network.

Communicating with Healthcare Providers

Effective communication with your healthcare team is essential for managing Exocrine Pancreatic Insufficiency (EPI) and optimizing your health and well-being. Establishing open, honest, and collaborative communication channels with your healthcare providers ensures that your needs are understood, your questions are addressed, and your treatment plan is tailored to your individual needs.

Preparing for Medical Appointments:

Before your medical appointments, take some time to prepare questions, concerns, and any relevant information you wish to discuss with your healthcare provider. Consider keeping a journal or diary to track your symptoms, dietary habits, medication adherence, and any changes in your condition since your last appointment. Bringing along a list of medications, supplements, and previous test results can also be helpful for your healthcare provider to gain a comprehensive understanding of your health status.

Active Participation in Discussions:

During your medical appointments, actively participate in discussions with your healthcare provider. Be honest and forthcoming about your symptoms, concerns, and preferences, and don't hesitate to ask questions or seek clarification on any aspects of your condition or treatment plan that you may not fully understand. Your healthcare provider is there to support you and provide guidance, so don't be afraid to speak up and advocate for your needs.

Seeking Clarification and Understanding:

If you're unsure about a particular aspect of your diagnosis, treatment plan, or recommended lifestyle adjustments, don't hesitate to seek clarification from your healthcare provider. Ask for explanations in plain language, and request additional information or resources if needed to help you better understand your condition and the rationale behind your treatment recommendations. Understanding your condition empowers you to take an active role in managing it effectively.

Discussing Treatment Options and Preferences:

Be proactive in discussing treatment options and preferences with your healthcare provider. Share your goals, preferences, and concerns regarding treatment, and work collaboratively to develop a treatment plan that aligns with your individual needs and priorities. Your healthcare provider can offer insights into available treatment options, potential benefits and risks, and alternative approaches to managing your condition.

Following Up and Providing Feedback:

After your medical appointments, follow up with your healthcare provider as needed to address any lingering questions or concerns, provide updates on your condition, and discuss the effectiveness of your treatment plan. Provide feedback on your experiences with treatment, including any side effects, challenges, or improvements you've noticed, to help your healthcare provider tailor your care plan and optimize your outcomes.

Utilizing Telemedicine and Remote Communication:

In today's digital age, telemedicine and remote communication technologies offer convenient ways to connect with your healthcare provider, particularly for routine check-ups, follow-up appointments, and minor concerns. Take advantage of telemedicine services when appropriate to maintain regular contact with your healthcare team and receive timely support and guidance without the need for in-person visits.

CHAPTER 3

THE EPI DIET: FOUNDATION FOR WELLNESS

The EPI diet plays a crucial role in managing Exocrine Pancreatic Insufficiency (EPI) and optimizing digestive health and overall well-being. This chapter explores the principles of the EPI diet, dietary strategies to support digestive function, and practical tips for meal planning, food selection, and nutritional supplementation.

Understanding the EPI Diet:

The EPI diet is designed to support individuals with EPI in optimizing nutrient absorption, minimizing digestive discomfort, and maintaining overall health and well-being. It focuses on selecting foods that are easily digestible, low in fat, and rich in essential nutrients, while avoiding foods that may exacerbate symptoms or strain the digestive system.

Key Principles of the EPI Diet:

1. **Moderate Fat Intake:** Limiting dietary fat is essential for individuals with EPI, as impaired fat digestion is a hallmark feature of the condition. Choose lean protein sources, minimize added fats and oils, and opt for cooking methods such as baking, grilling, or steaming rather than frying.

2. **High Protein Content:** Protein is vital for supporting muscle strength, immune function, and tissue repair, making it an important component of the EPI diet. Include lean sources of

protein in your meals, such as poultry, fish, tofu, legumes, and low-fat dairy products.

3. **Complex Carbohydrates:** Carbohydrates provide energy and fiber, which are essential for digestive health and overall well-being. Choose complex carbohydrates such as whole grains, fruits, vegetables, and legumes, which provide sustained energy and promote satiety.

4. **Fiber-Rich Foods:** Fiber promotes regularity, aids in digestion, and supports gut health. Incorporate fiber-rich foods into your diet, such as fruits, vegetables, whole grains, nuts, seeds, and legumes, while being mindful of your individual tolerance levels.

Practical Tips for Meal Planning:

1. **Small, Frequent Meals:** Eating smaller, more frequent meals throughout the day can help prevent digestive overload and minimize symptoms of bloating, gas, and discomfort.

2. **Balanced Plate Method:** Aim to include a balance of protein, carbohydrates, and healthy fats in each meal to support balanced nutrition and optimal digestion.

3. **Food Selection:** Choose foods that are easily digestible and well-tolerated, such as cooked vegetables, lean proteins, whole grains, and low-fat dairy products. Experiment with different foods to identify your individual triggers and preferences.

4. **Hydration:** Stay hydrated by drinking plenty of water throughout the day, as adequate hydration is essential for supporting digestive function and overall health.

Nutritional Supplementation:

In addition to dietary modifications, nutritional supplementation may be recommended to address specific nutrient deficiencies or support digestive function. Your healthcare provider or dietitian may recommend enzyme replacement therapy, vitamin and mineral supplements, or specialized nutritional formulas to optimize your nutritional status and overall well-being.

Seeking Guidance from a Dietitian:

Consulting with a registered dietitian or nutritionist who specializes in digestive health can provide personalized guidance and support in implementing the EPI diet. A dietitian can help you develop a tailored meal plan, address dietary concerns and preferences, and monitor your nutritional status to ensure optimal health and well-being.

Principles of the EPI Diet

The EPI diet is designed to support individuals with Exocrine Pancreatic Insufficiency (EPI) in optimizing nutrient absorption, minimizing digestive discomfort, and maintaining overall health and well-being. It emphasizes dietary strategies that promote efficient digestion, enhance nutrient absorption, and reduce the risk of gastrointestinal symptoms.

1. Moderate Fat Intake:

Individuals with EPI often have difficulty digesting fats due to insufficient pancreatic enzyme production. Therefore, the EPI diet typically includes moderate fat intake, focusing on sources of healthy fats that are easier to digest, such as monounsaturated and polyunsaturated fats. Limiting dietary fat can help prevent symptoms such as bloating, gas, and diarrhea associated with fat malabsorption.

2. Emphasis on Lean Proteins:

Protein is essential for supporting muscle function, immune health, and tissue repair, making it a crucial component of the EPI diet. Lean protein sources, such as poultry, fish, tofu, legumes, and low-fat dairy products, are preferred, as they provide essential amino acids without adding excessive fat or strain on the digestive system.

3. Complex Carbohydrates:

Carbohydrates are a primary source of energy for the body and play a crucial role in supporting digestive health and overall well-being. The EPI diet emphasizes complex carbohydrates, such as whole grains, fruits, vegetables, and legumes, which provide sustained energy, fiber, vitamins, and minerals. These nutrient-rich carbohydrates support digestive function and promote satiety.

4. Fiber-Rich Foods:

Fiber is essential for promoting regularity, supporting gut health, and preventing constipation, which can be common symptoms of EPI. Including fiber-rich foods in the EPI diet, such as fruits, vegetables, whole grains, nuts, seeds, and legumes, helps maintain healthy bowel function and supports optimal digestion. However, individuals with EPI should be mindful of their individual tolerance to fiber and adjust their intake accordingly to prevent digestive discomfort.

5. Hydration:

Proper hydration is essential for supporting digestive function, nutrient absorption, and overall health. Drinking an adequate amount of water throughout the day helps maintain hydration, supports bowel regularity, and aids in the digestion and absorption of nutrients. Individuals with EPI should aim to drink plenty of water and hydrating fluids to support optimal digestive health and well-being.

6. Individualized Approach:

The EPI diet is not one-size-fits-all, and individual dietary needs and preferences may vary. It's essential to take an individualized approach to the EPI diet, considering factors such as personal taste, cultural background, food tolerances, and nutritional requirements. Working with a registered dietitian or nutritionist can help individuals tailor their diet to their specific needs and preferences while ensuring optimal nutritional intake and digestive health.

Essential Nutrients for EPI Management

Managing Exocrine Pancreatic Insufficiency (EPI) requires careful attention to nutritional intake to ensure adequate nutrient absorption, support digestive function, and maintain overall health and well-being. Certain nutrients play a particularly important role in EPI management, and focusing on these essential nutrients can help individuals optimize their nutritional status and minimize symptoms associated with the condition.

1. Digestive Enzymes:

One of the hallmark features of EPI is insufficient production or secretion of digestive enzymes by the pancreas. As a result, individuals with EPI often require enzyme replacement therapy to aid in the digestion and absorption of nutrients. Pancreatic enzyme supplements, which contain enzymes such as lipase, protease, and amylase, are taken with meals to help break down fats, proteins, and carbohydrates and facilitate nutrient absorption.

2. Fat-Soluble Vitamins:

Fat malabsorption is a common complication of EPI, leading to deficiencies in fat-soluble vitamins such as vitamin A, D, E, and K. These vitamins play essential roles in various physiological processes, including immune function, bone health, vision, and blood clotting. Individuals with EPI may require supplementation with fat-soluble vitamins to prevent deficiencies and maintain optimal health.

3. Water-Soluble Vitamins:

In addition to fat-soluble vitamins, individuals with EPI may also be at risk of deficiencies in water-soluble vitamins, such as vitamin B12 and folate. These vitamins play crucial roles in energy metabolism, nerve function, red blood cell production, and DNA synthesis. Supplementation with water-soluble vitamins may be necessary to ensure adequate intake and prevent deficiencies in individuals with EPI.

4. Minerals:

EPI can also lead to deficiencies in essential minerals, such as calcium, magnesium, and zinc, which are important for bone health, muscle function, and immune support. Individuals with EPI may require supplementation with minerals to maintain optimal levels and prevent deficiencies. Calcium and magnesium supplements may also help alleviate symptoms of muscle cramps and bone pain associated with EPI-related malabsorption.

5. Protein-Rich Foods:

Protein is vital for supporting muscle strength, immune function, and tissue repair, making it an essential nutrient for individuals with EPI. Lean protein sources, such as poultry, fish, tofu, legumes, and low-fat dairy products, are preferred, as they provide essential amino acids without adding excessive fat or strain on the digestive system.

6. Fluids and Electrolytes:

Dehydration and electrolyte imbalances can occur as a result of EPI-related diarrhea and fluid loss. It's essential for individuals with EPI to stay hydrated by drinking plenty of water and electrolyte-rich fluids, such as sports drinks or oral rehydration solutions, to maintain fluid and electrolyte balance and prevent dehydration.

Tailoring Your Diet to Your Needs

While there are general principles to follow when it comes to the EPI diet, it's essential to tailor your dietary approach to your individual needs, preferences, and tolerances. By taking a personalized approach to your diet, you can optimize nutrient intake, manage symptoms, and enhance overall well-being while living with Exocrine Pancreatic Insufficiency (EPI).

1. Identify Trigger Foods:

Keep track of your dietary intake and symptoms to identify trigger foods that may exacerbate digestive symptoms or discomfort. Common trigger foods for individuals with EPI may include high-fat foods, spicy foods, greasy foods, dairy products, and certain types of fiber-rich foods. By identifying and avoiding trigger foods, you can minimize symptoms and promote digestive comfort.

2. Experiment with Food Preparation Methods:

Experiment with different food preparation methods to determine which ones are most easily digestible and well-tolerated for you. Cooking methods such as baking, grilling, steaming, and poaching are often gentler on the digestive system than frying or sautéing. Choose cooking techniques that help retain the nutritional integrity of foods while making them easier to digest.

3. Consider Meal Timing and Frequency:

Pay attention to your meal timing and frequency to prevent digestive overload and minimize symptoms such as bloating, gas, and discomfort. Eating smaller, more frequent meals throughout the day can help regulate blood sugar levels, support digestion, and prevent symptoms associated with large meals. Experiment with meal timing and frequency to find a pattern that works best for your individual needs.

4. Focus on Nutrient-Dense Foods:

Prioritize nutrient-dense foods that provide essential vitamins, minerals, and antioxidants to support overall health and well-being. Include a variety of fruits, vegetables, whole grains, lean proteins, and healthy fats in your diet to ensure a diverse range of nutrients and promote optimal nutrition. Nutrient-dense foods can help meet your nutritional needs while minimizing digestive strain.

5. Work with a Registered Dietitian:

Consulting with a registered dietitian or nutritionist who specializes in digestive health can provide personalized guidance and support in tailoring your diet to your specific needs. A dietitian can help you develop a customized meal plan, address dietary concerns and preferences, and monitor your nutritional status to ensure optimal health and well-being. Working with a dietitian empowers you to make informed dietary choices and achieve your health goals.

6. Listen to Your Body:

Above all, listen to your body and honor its cues and signals regarding hunger, fullness, and satisfaction. Pay attention to how different foods and eating patterns affect your digestion, energy levels, and overall well-being. By tuning into your body's needs and preferences, you can make dietary choices that support optimal health and quality of life while living with EPI.

CHAPTER 4

NAVIGATING NUTRITION WITH EPI

Living with Exocrine Pancreatic Insufficiency (EPI) presents unique challenges when it comes to nutrition and dietary management. This chapter explores strategies for navigating nutrition with EPI, including meal planning, dietary modifications, nutritional supplementation, and lifestyle adjustments to optimize digestive health and overall well-being.

Understanding the Role of Nutrition:

Nutrition plays a critical role in managing EPI and supporting overall health and well-being. A well-balanced diet provides essential nutrients, supports digestive function, and helps prevent complications associated with EPI, such as malnutrition, weight loss, and gastrointestinal symptoms. By understanding the role of nutrition in managing EPI, individuals can make informed dietary choices to support their health and quality of life.

Meal Planning for EPI:

Meal planning is essential for individuals with EPI to ensure they receive adequate nutrition while minimizing digestive discomfort. By focusing on nutrient-dense foods, portion control, and meal timing, individuals can optimize digestion, support nutrient absorption, and prevent symptoms associated with EPI. Meal planning strategies may include smaller, more frequent meals, balanced plate composition, and consideration of individual dietary preferences and tolerances.

Dietary Modifications for EPI:

Dietary modifications may be necessary for individuals with EPI to manage symptoms and support digestive health. Common dietary modifications for EPI may include limiting dietary fat, avoiding trigger foods, incorporating enzyme-rich foods, and emphasizing easily digestible foods. By making targeted dietary modifications, individuals can minimize symptoms and optimize their nutritional intake while living with EPI.

Nutritional Supplementation:

Nutritional supplementation plays a crucial role in managing EPI-related nutrient deficiencies and supporting overall health and well-being. Individuals with EPI may require supplementation with digestive enzymes, vitamins, minerals, and other nutrients to address specific nutritional needs and prevent complications associated with EPI. Working with a healthcare provider or dietitian can help individuals identify appropriate supplements and optimize their nutritional status.

Lifestyle Adjustments:

In addition to dietary modifications and supplementation, lifestyle adjustments can further support digestive health and overall well-being for individuals with EPI. Lifestyle adjustments may include stress management techniques, regular physical activity, adequate hydration, and avoiding smoking and excessive alcohol consumption. By incorporating healthy lifestyle habits into their daily routine, individuals can enhance the effectiveness of their EPI management plan and improve their quality of life.

Seeking Support and Guidance:

Navigating nutrition with EPI can be challenging, but individuals don't have to do it alone. Seeking support and guidance from healthcare providers, dietitians, support groups, and online communities can provide valuable resources, information, and encouragement for managing EPI and optimizing nutrition. By building a supportive network of healthcare professionals and peers, individuals can gain confidence, knowledge, and empowerment in managing their condition effectively.

Understanding Enzyme Replacement Therapy (ERT)

Enzyme Replacement Therapy (ERT) is a cornerstone of treatment for individuals with Exocrine Pancreatic Insufficiency (EPI). This section explores the role of ERT in managing EPI, how it works, administration methods, dosage considerations, and potential benefits and side effects.

Role of Enzyme Replacement Therapy:

ERT is designed to supplement the deficient pancreatic enzymes in individuals with EPI, aiding in the digestion and absorption of nutrients from food. By providing exogenous enzymes in the form of oral capsules or tablets, ERT helps compensate for the insufficient enzyme production by the pancreas, thereby improving digestive function and alleviating symptoms associated with EPI.

Mechanism of Action:

Pancreatic enzymes, such as lipase, protease, and amylase, play a crucial role in breaking down fats, proteins, and carbohydrates in the digestive tract. In individuals with EPI, the pancreas fails to produce an adequate amount of these enzymes, leading to impaired digestion and nutrient malabsorption. ERT supplements provide these missing enzymes, facilitating the breakdown of nutrients and promoting optimal absorption.

Administration Methods:

ERT is typically administered orally in the form of enteric-coated capsules or tablets, which are designed to resist degradation by stomach acid and release the enzymes in the alkaline environment of the small intestine. The capsules or tablets are taken with meals and snacks to coincide with food ingestion, allowing the enzymes to mix with the food bolus and facilitate digestion.

Dosage Considerations:

The dosage of ERT is individualized based on factors such as the severity of EPI, the patient's nutritional status, dietary intake, and response to treatment. Healthcare providers may adjust the dosage of ERT based on symptoms, stool consistency, nutritional markers, and imaging studies. It's essential for individuals with EPI to follow their healthcare provider's recommendations regarding ERT dosage and administration for optimal efficacy.

Benefits of ERT:

ERT offers several benefits for individuals with EPI, including improved digestion, enhanced nutrient absorption, reduction of gastrointestinal symptoms such as bloating, gas, and diarrhea, and prevention of EPI-related complications such as malnutrition and weight loss. By addressing the underlying enzyme deficiency, ERT helps individuals with EPI maintain nutritional balance and improve their quality of life.

Potential Side Effects:

While ERT is generally well-tolerated, some individuals may experience side effects such as abdominal pain, bloating, gas, nausea, and diarrhea, especially during the initial phase of treatment or with higher doses. These side effects are usually mild and transient and can often be managed by adjusting the dosage of ERT or taking the enzymes with different meals.

Conclusion:

Enzyme Replacement Therapy (ERT) is an essential component of treatment for individuals with Exocrine Pancreatic Insufficiency (EPI), providing exogenous pancreatic enzymes to support digestion and nutrient absorption. By understanding the role, mechanism of action, administration methods, dosage considerations, benefits, and potential side effects of ERT, individuals with EPI can effectively manage their condition and improve their digestive health and overall well-being.

Optimizing Enzyme Use with Meals and Snacks

Ensuring optimal timing and dosage of enzyme replacement therapy (ERT) is crucial for individuals with Exocrine Pancreatic Insufficiency (EPI) to maximize its effectiveness and promote efficient digestion. This section explores strategies for optimizing enzyme use with meals and snacks, including timing, dosage, and considerations for various types of foods.

Timing of Enzyme Administration:

Taking pancreatic enzyme supplements at the right time is essential for maximizing their effectiveness in aiding digestion. Ideally, enzymes should be taken just before or at the beginning of meals and snacks to ensure they mix with the food bolus and facilitate digestion throughout the digestive tract. By timing enzyme administration with food intake, individuals can enhance nutrient absorption and minimize digestive discomfort.

Dosage Considerations:

Determining the appropriate dosage of pancreatic enzymes depends on factors such as the individual's pancreatic enzyme output, the fat content of the meal or snack, and the severity of EPI symptoms. Healthcare providers may recommend adjusting the dosage of enzymes based on these factors to ensure optimal digestion and symptom management. It's essential for individuals with EPI to follow their healthcare provider's guidance regarding enzyme dosage and administration for optimal results.

Matching Enzyme Dosage to Meal Composition:

Tailoring enzyme dosage to the composition of meals and snacks can help optimize digestion and nutrient absorption for individuals with EPI. Higher fat meals may require a higher dosage of enzymes to ensure adequate fat digestion, while lower fat meals may require a lower dosage. By matching enzyme dosage to meal composition, individuals can optimize digestion and prevent symptoms associated with EPI-related malabsorption.

Considerations for Different Types of Foods:

Certain types of foods may require special considerations when it comes to enzyme use and digestion. For example, fatty foods may require a higher dosage of enzymes to facilitate fat digestion, while high-fiber foods may require enzymes with additional protease to break down plant-based fibers. Individuals with EPI should work with their healthcare provider or dietitian to determine the appropriate enzyme dosage and formulation for their dietary needs and preferences.

Monitoring and Adjusting:

Regular monitoring of symptoms, stool consistency, and nutritional markers can help individuals with EPI assess the effectiveness of enzyme replacement therapy and make necessary adjustments to optimize digestion and symptom management. Healthcare providers may recommend periodic evaluations and adjustments to enzyme dosage based on the individual's response to treatment and changes in dietary intake or symptoms.

Conclusion:

Optimizing enzyme use with meals and snacks is essential for individuals with Exocrine Pancreatic Insufficiency (EPI) to maximize the effectiveness of enzyme replacement therapy (ERT) and promote efficient digestion. By timing enzyme administration, adjusting dosage based on meal composition, and monitoring symptoms, individuals with EPI can optimize their digestive health and overall well-being.

Exploring Dietary Supplements

In addition to enzyme replacement therapy (ERT), individuals with Exocrine Pancreatic Insufficiency (EPI) may benefit from dietary supplements to address specific nutritional needs, support digestive function, and optimize overall health and well-being. This section explores common dietary supplements used in EPI management, their roles, benefits, and considerations for use.

1. Fat-Soluble Vitamins:

Fat malabsorption is a common complication of EPI, leading to deficiencies in fat-soluble vitamins such as vitamin A, D, E, and K. Supplementation with fat-soluble vitamins can help prevent deficiencies and support various physiological processes, including immune function, bone health, vision, and blood clotting. Healthcare providers may recommend vitamin supplementation based on individual nutritional needs and blood test results.

2. Water-Soluble Vitamins:

In addition to fat-soluble vitamins, individuals with EPI may also be at risk of deficiencies in water-soluble vitamins, such as vitamin B12 and folate. Supplementation with water-soluble vitamins can help address deficiencies and support energy metabolism, nerve function, red blood cell production, and DNA synthesis. Healthcare providers may prescribe vitamin supplements based on individual nutritional status and dietary intake.

3. Minerals:

EPI-related malabsorption can also lead to deficiencies in essential minerals, such as calcium, magnesium, and zinc, which are important for bone health, muscle function, and immune support. Supplementation with minerals can help maintain optimal mineral levels and prevent deficiencies in individuals with EPI. Healthcare providers may recommend mineral supplements based on individual nutritional needs and blood test results.

4. Digestive Enzymes:

While enzyme replacement therapy (ERT) is the primary treatment for EPI, some individuals may benefit from additional digestive enzyme supplements to support digestion and alleviate symptoms. Supplemental enzymes containing lipase, protease, and amylase can help further break down nutrients from food and promote optimal absorption. Healthcare providers may recommend digestive enzyme supplements based on individual symptoms and response to treatment.

5. Probiotics:

Probiotics are beneficial bacteria that support digestive health by promoting a healthy balance of gut microflora and enhancing immune function. Individuals with EPI may experience alterations in gut microbiota due to malabsorption and digestive disturbances. Supplementing with probiotics may help restore gut health and alleviate symptoms such as bloating, gas, and diarrhea. Healthcare providers may recommend specific probiotic strains and formulations based on individual needs and symptoms.

6. Omega-3 Fatty Acids:

Omega-3 fatty acids, found in fatty fish, flaxseeds, and walnuts, have anti-inflammatory properties and may help reduce inflammation and improve digestive health in individuals with EPI. Supplementing with omega-3 fatty acids can support cardiovascular health, reduce inflammation in the digestive tract, and promote overall well-being. Healthcare providers may recommend omega-3 supplements as part of a comprehensive EPI management plan.

Conclusion:

Dietary supplements play a valuable role in supporting digestive health, addressing nutritional deficiencies, and optimizing overall well-being for individuals with Exocrine Pancreatic Insufficiency (EPI). By exploring the use of dietary supplements under the guidance of healthcare providers, individuals with EPI can enhance their nutritional status, manage symptoms, and improve their quality of life.

CHAPTER 5

THE EPI COOKBOOK: ESSENTIAL RECIPES AND MEAL PLANS

This chapter serves as a practical guide for individuals with Exocrine Pancreatic Insufficiency (EPI) to navigate their dietary needs with delicious and nutritious recipes and meal plans. From breakfast to dinner, snacks to desserts, each recipe is carefully crafted to be gentle on the digestive system while providing essential nutrients and flavors to support overall well-being.

Introduction to the EPI Cookbook:

The EPI Cookbook is more than just a collection of recipes; it's a resource designed to empower individuals with EPI to enjoy delicious and satisfying meals while managing their condition effectively. Whether you're newly diagnosed or a seasoned EPI warrior, these recipes and meal plans are tailored to your dietary needs and preferences.

Navigating the EPI Diet:

Before diving into the recipes and meal plans, it's essential to understand the principles of the EPI diet and how to adapt them to your individual needs. From choosing enzyme-friendly ingredients to balancing macronutrients, this section provides guidance on navigating the EPI diet with confidence and creativity.

Essential Recipes for EPI Management:

Explore a variety of essential recipes designed specifically for individuals with EPI, including:

1. **Enzyme-Friendly Breakfasts:** Start your day right with delicious and nutritious breakfast options that are easy on the digestive system, such as oatmeal, smoothies, and scrambled eggs with toast.

2. **Gut-Healing Soups and Stews:** Warm up with comforting soups and stews packed with flavor and nutrients, such as chicken noodle soup, vegetable broth, and lentil stew.

3. **Enzyme-Friendly Entrées:** Enjoy satisfying entrées that are gentle on the digestive system, such as baked chicken, grilled fish, tofu stir-fry, and quinoa salad.

4. **Enzyme-Friendly Sides:** Complement your meals with flavorful side dishes that support digestion and provide essential nutrients, such as roasted vegetables, steamed rice, and mashed potatoes.

5. **Healthy Snacks and Treats:** Indulge in nutritious snacks and treats that satisfy cravings without compromising digestive health, such as fruit smoothies, yogurt parfaits, and homemade energy balls.

Meal Plans for EPI Wellness:

In addition to individual recipes, this chapter includes sample meal plans designed to help you plan your meals and snacks for the week ahead. Each meal plan is carefully curated to provide balanced nutrition, variety, and flexibility while accommodating the dietary needs of individuals with EPI.

Cooking Tips and Techniques:

Enhance your culinary skills with cooking tips and techniques specifically tailored to individuals with EPI. Learn how to modify recipes to make them more enzyme-friendly, choose cooking methods that support digestion, and experiment with flavor combinations to create delicious and nutritious meals.

Conclusion:

The EPI Cookbook is your go-to resource for delicious and nutritious recipes and meal plans designed to support digestive health and overall well-being. By incorporating enzyme-friendly ingredients, balanced nutrition, and creative cooking techniques into your meals, you can enjoy a diverse and satisfying diet while managing your EPI effectively.

Breakfasts for Digestive Ease

Starting your day with a nourishing and enzyme-friendly breakfast sets the tone for optimal digestion and overall well-being. This section offers a variety of breakfast recipes designed to be gentle on the digestive system while providing essential nutrients and energy to kickstart your morning.

1. Oatmeal with Berries and Almonds:

- **Ingredients**:
    - Rolled oats
    - Almond milk
    - Fresh berries (e.g., strawberries, blueberries, raspberries)

- Sliced almonds
- Honey or maple syrup (optional)

- **Instructions:**
  - Cook rolled oats according to package instructions with almond milk for added creaminess.
  - Top with fresh berries and sliced almonds for added flavor and texture.
  - Drizzle with honey or maple syrup if desired for sweetness.

2. Yogurt Parfait with Granola and Fruit:

- **Ingredients**:
  - Greek yogurt (or dairy-free alternative)
  - Granola (look for low-fat and low-sugar options)
  - Fresh fruit (e.g., bananas, kiwi, pineapple)
  - Honey or agave syrup (optional)

- **Instructions**:
  - Layer Greek yogurt, granola, and fresh fruit in a parfait glass or bowl.
  - Repeat layers until the glass is filled.
  - Drizzle with honey or agave syrup if desired for added sweetness.

3. **Scrambled Eggs with Spinach and Feta:**

   - **Ingredients:**
     - Eggs
     - Fresh spinach leaves
     - Crumbled feta cheese
     - Olive oil or butter

   - **Instructions:**
     - In a skillet, heat olive oil or butter over medium heat.
     - Add fresh spinach leaves and cook until wilted.
     - Whisk eggs in a bowl and pour into the skillet over the spinach.
     - Cook, stirring occasionally, until eggs are scrambled and cooked through.
     - Sprinkle with crumbled feta cheese before serving.

4. **Smoothie with Banana and Peanut Butter:**

   - **Ingredients:**
     - Ripe bananas
     - Peanut butter (or almond butter for a nut-free option)
     - Almond milk (or dairy-free alternative)
     - Spinach leaves (optional for added greens)

- **Instructions:**

  - Blend ripe bananas, peanut butter, almond milk, and spinach leaves (if using) until smooth and creamy.

  - Pour into a glass and enjoy as a refreshing and nutrient-packed breakfast smoothie.

5. Toast with Avocado and Tomato:

- **Ingredients:**

  - Whole grain bread (or gluten-free bread for a gluten-free option)

  - Ripe avocado

  - Sliced tomato

  - Sea salt and black pepper

- **Instructions:**

  - Toast whole grain bread until golden brown.

  - Mash ripe avocado onto the toasted bread and spread evenly.

  - Top with sliced tomato and season with sea salt and black pepper to taste.

Conclusion:

These enzyme-friendly breakfast recipes are designed to provide nourishment, energy, and digestive ease to individuals with Exocrine Pancreatic Insufficiency (EPI). By incorporating nutrient-rich ingredients and flavorful combinations into your morning routine, you can start your day on the right foot and support optimal digestive health.

Lunches to Fuel Your Day

Midday meals should provide sustained energy and nourishment to support you through the rest of your day. This section offers a variety of lunch recipes designed to be both satisfying and gentle on the digestive system, ensuring you stay fueled and focused until dinnertime.

1. Quinoa Salad with Roasted Vegetables:

- **Ingredients:**
    - Quinoa
    - Assorted vegetables (e.g., bell peppers, zucchini, cherry tomatoes)
    - Olive oil
    - Balsamic vinegar
    - Fresh herbs (e.g., parsley, basil)

- **Instructions:**
  - Cook quinoa according to package instructions and set aside to cool.
  - Chop assorted vegetables into bite-sized pieces and toss with olive oil.
  - Roast vegetables in the oven until tender and slightly caramelized.
  - In a large bowl, combine cooked quinoa, roasted vegetables, balsamic vinegar, and fresh herbs.
  - Toss gently to combine and serve as a nutritious and satisfying salad.

2. **Grilled Chicken Wrap with Hummus and Greens:**

- **Ingredients:**
  - Grilled chicken breast, sliced
  - Whole grain wrap (or gluten-free wrap for a gluten-free option)
  - Hummus
  - Mixed greens (e.g., spinach, arugula)
  - Sliced cucumber and tomato

- **Instructions:**
  - Lay a whole grain wrap flat and spread a generous layer of hummus over it.
  - Layer sliced grilled chicken breast, mixed greens, sliced cucumber, and tomato on top of the hummus.
  - Roll up the wrap tightly, slice in half, and enjoy as a satisfying and protein-packed lunch option.

3. Lentil Soup with Spinach and Carrots:

- **Ingredients:**
  - Dried lentils
  - Onion, diced
  - Carrots, diced
  - Fresh spinach leaves
  - Vegetable broth
  - Garlic, minced

- **Instructions:**
  - In a large pot, sauté diced onion and minced garlic until fragrant.
  - Add diced carrots and dried lentils to the pot, along with vegetable broth.
  - Simmer until lentils are tender and soup has thickened.

- Stir in fresh spinach leaves just before serving and season with salt and pepper to taste.

4. **Tofu Stir-Fry with Brown Rice:**

- **Ingredients:**
  - Extra-firm tofu, cubed
  - Assorted vegetables (e.g., bell peppers, broccoli, snap peas)
  - Soy sauce (or tamari for a gluten-free option)
  - Sesame oil
  - Cooked brown rice

- **Instructions:**
  - In a large skillet or wok, heat sesame oil over medium-high heat.
  - Add cubed tofu to the skillet and cook until golden brown on all sides.
  - Add assorted vegetables to the skillet and stir-fry until tender-crisp.
  - Drizzle with soy sauce or tamari and toss to coat.
  - Serve tofu stir-fry over cooked brown rice for a satisfying and nutritious lunch.

5. Quinoa and Black Bean Salad with Avocado Dressing:

- **Ingredients:**
    - Cooked quinoa
    - Black beans, drained and rinsed
    - Ripe avocado
    - Lime juice
    - Cilantro
- **Instructions:**
    - In a large bowl, combine cooked quinoa and black beans.
    - Mash ripe avocado with lime juice and chopped cilantro to make a creamy dressing.
    - Toss quinoa and black bean salad with avocado dressing until well coated.
    - Serve chilled or at room temperature as a flavorful and protein-rich salad option.

Conclusion:

These lunch recipes are designed to provide sustained energy, nourishment, and satisfaction for individuals with Exocrine Pancreatic Insufficiency (EPI). By incorporating nutrient-dense ingredients and flavorful combinations into your midday meals, you can fuel your day and support optimal digestive health.

Dinners for Digestive Delight

Evening meals should be satisfying and comforting while remaining gentle on the digestive system. This section offers a variety of dinner recipes designed to be flavorful, nutritious, and easy to digest, ensuring a delightful dining experience for individuals with Exocrine Pancreatic Insufficiency (EPI).

1. Baked Salmon with Lemon and Herbs:

- **Ingredients:**
    - Salmon fillets
    - Fresh lemon slices
    - Fresh herbs (e.g., dill, parsley)
    - Olive oil
- **Instructions:**
    - Preheat oven to 375°F (190°C) and line a baking sheet with parchment paper.
    - Place salmon fillets on the prepared baking sheet and drizzle with olive oil.
    - Season with fresh lemon slices and chopped herbs.

- Bake in the preheated oven for 15-20 minutes, or until salmon is cooked through and flakes easily with a fork.

2. Vegetable Stir-Fry with Tofu:

- **Ingredients:**
  - Extra-firm tofu, cubed
  - Assorted vegetables (e.g., bell peppers, broccoli, carrots)
  - Soy sauce (or tamari for a gluten-free option)
  - Sesame oil

- **Instructions:**
  - In a large skillet or wok, heat sesame oil over medium-high heat.
  - Add cubed tofu to the skillet and cook until golden brown on all sides.
  - Add assorted vegetables to the skillet and stir-fry until tender-crisp.
  - Drizzle with soy sauce or tamari and toss to coat.
  - Serve vegetable stir-fry over cooked brown rice or quinoa for a satisfying and nutritious dinner.

3. Turkey Meatballs with Marinara Sauce:

- **Ingredients:**
  - Ground turkey

- Breadcrumbs (or gluten-free breadcrumbs for a gluten-free option)
- Egg
- Italian seasoning
- Marinara sauce (look for low-fat and low-sugar options)

- **Instructions:**
  - In a mixing bowl, combine ground turkey, breadcrumbs, egg, and Italian seasoning.
  - Form mixture into meatballs and place on a baking sheet lined with parchment paper.
  - Bake in a preheated oven at 375°F (190°C) for 20-25 minutes, or until meatballs are cooked through.
  - Serve turkey meatballs with marinara sauce over cooked whole grain pasta or zucchini noodles.

4. **Vegetable Curry with Chickpeas:**

- **Ingredients:**
  - Chickpeas, drained and rinsed
  - Assorted vegetables (e.g., cauliflower, bell peppers, peas)
  - Curry powder
  - Coconut milk

- **Instructions:**
  - In a large pot, combine chickpeas, assorted vegetables, curry powder, and coconut milk.
  - Simmer over medium heat until vegetables are tender and curry is fragrant.
  - Serve vegetable curry over cooked brown rice or quinoa for a flavorful and satisfying dinner option.

5. **Grilled Chicken Salad with Avocado Dressing:**

- **Ingredients:**
  - Grilled chicken breast, sliced
  - Mixed salad greens (e.g., spinach, arugula, romaine)
  - Cherry tomatoes, halved
  - Sliced cucumber
  - Avocado

- **Instructions:**
  - Arrange mixed salad greens, cherry tomatoes, and sliced cucumber on a serving plate.
  - Top with grilled chicken breast slices and sliced avocado.
  - Drizzle with avocado dressing or your favorite vinaigrette.

Conclusion:

These dinner recipes are designed to provide flavorful, nutritious, and easy-to-digest options for individuals with Exocrine Pancreatic Insufficiency (EPI). By incorporating wholesome ingredients and simple cooking techniques, you can enjoy delicious and satisfying meals while supporting optimal digestive health.

Snacks and Treats for Every Craving

Snacking can be a delightful way to satisfy cravings and keep energy levels up throughout the day. This section offers a variety of snack and treat recipes designed to be both delicious and gentle on the digestive system, ensuring you can indulge without discomfort.

1. Fruit and Nut Energy Balls:

- **Ingredients:**
    - Medjool dates, pitted
    - Almonds
    - Rolled oats
    - Unsweetened shredded coconut
    - Cocoa powder

- **Instructions:**
  - In a food processor, combine pitted dates, almonds, rolled oats, shredded coconut, and cocoa powder.
  - Pulse until mixture comes together and forms a sticky dough.
  - Roll mixture into small balls and place on a baking sheet lined with parchment paper.
  - Refrigerate for at least 30 minutes to firm up before serving.

2. Greek Yogurt Parfait with Berries:

- **Ingredients:**
  - Greek yogurt (or dairy-free alternative)
  - Fresh berries (e.g., strawberries, blueberries, raspberries)
  - Granola

- **Instructions:**
  - Layer Greek yogurt, fresh berries, and granola in a parfait glass or bowl.
  - Repeat layers until the glass is filled.
  - Serve chilled as a satisfying and protein-rich snack or dessert option.

3. **Hummus and Veggie Crudité:**

   - **Ingredients:**
     - Hummus
     - Assorted raw vegetables (e.g., carrots, cucumber, bell peppers)
   - **Instructions:**
     - Cut raw vegetables into bite-sized pieces and arrange on a serving platter.
     - Serve with hummus for dipping for a crunchy and satisfying snack option.

4. **Peanut Butter Banana Smoothie:**

   - **Ingredients:**
     - Ripe bananas
     - Peanut butter (or almond butter for a nut-free option)
     - Almond milk (or dairy-free alternative)
     - Ice cubes
   - **Instructions:**
     - Blend ripe bananas, peanut butter, almond milk, and ice cubes until smooth and creamy.
     - Pour into a glass and enjoy as a refreshing and satisfying snack or dessert option.

5. Rice Cake with Avocado and Tomato:

- **Ingredients:**
    - Rice cakes (or gluten-free rice cakes for a gluten-free option)
    - Ripe avocado
    - Sliced tomato
    - Sea salt and black pepper
- **Instructions**:
    - Spread ripe avocado onto rice cakes and top with sliced tomato.
    - Season with sea salt and black pepper to taste for a crunchy and savory snack option.

Conclusion:

These snack and treat recipes offer a variety of options to satisfy cravings and keep energy levels up throughout the day for individuals with Exocrine Pancreatic Insufficiency (EPI). By incorporating nutrient-rich ingredients and wholesome flavors into your snacks and treats, you can indulge without discomfort and support optimal digestive health.

Sample Meal Plans for Different Dietary Preferences

Meal planning can simplify the process of eating well and managing Exocrine Pancreatic Insufficiency (EPI). This section offers a variety of sample meal plans tailored to different dietary preferences, ensuring there's something for everyone to enjoy while supporting optimal digestive health.

1. Balanced Meal Plan:

- Breakfast: Oatmeal with Berries and Almonds
- Lunch: Grilled Chicken Wrap with Hummus and Greens
- Dinner: Baked Salmon with Lemon and Herbs
- Snack: Greek Yogurt Parfait with Berries

2. Plant-Based Meal Plan:

- Breakfast: Smoothie with Banana and Peanut Butter
- Lunch: Vegetable Stir-Fry with Tofu
- Dinner: Vegetable Curry with Chickpeas
- Snack: Hummus and Veggie Crudité

3. Gluten-Free Meal Plan:

- Breakfast: Scrambled Eggs with Spinach and Feta
- Lunch: Turkey Meatballs with Marinara Sauce
- Dinner: Grilled Chicken Salad with Avocado Dressing
- Snack: Rice Cake with Avocado and Tomato

4. High-Protein Meal Plan:

- Breakfast: Greek Yogurt Parfait with Granola and Fruit
- Lunch: Lentil Soup with Spinach and Carrots
- Dinner: Turkey Meatballs with Marinara Sauce
- Snack: Fruit and Nut Energy Balls

5. Low-Carb Meal Plan:

- Breakfast: Scrambled Eggs with Spinach and Feta
- Lunch: Grilled Chicken Salad with Avocado Dressing
- Dinner: Baked Salmon with Lemon and Herbs
- Snack: Greek Yogurt Parfait with Berries

Conclusion:

These sample meal plans offer a variety of options to suit different dietary preferences while supporting optimal digestive health for individuals with Exocrine Pancreatic Insufficiency (EPI). Whether you prefer balanced, plant-based, gluten-free, high-protein, or low-carb meals, there are delicious and satisfying options to enjoy while managing EPI.

CHAPTER 6

LIFESTYLE STRATEGIES FOR EPI MANAGEMENT

Living well with Exocrine Pancreatic Insufficiency (EPI) involves more than just dietary adjustments. This chapter explores various lifestyle strategies and practical tips to enhance overall well-being and effectively manage EPI on a day-to-day basis.

1. Stress Management:

- Explore stress-reducing techniques such as meditation, deep breathing exercises, yoga, or tai chi to help manage stress levels, as stress can exacerbate digestive symptoms associated with EPI.

2. Physical Activity:

- Incorporate regular physical activity into your routine, such as walking, jogging, cycling, or swimming, to support digestive health and overall well-being. Aim for at least 30 minutes of moderate-intensity exercise most days of the week.

3. Hydration:

- Stay hydrated by drinking an adequate amount of water throughout the day. Aim for at least 8-10 glasses of water daily to support digestion and prevent dehydration, which can worsen gastrointestinal symptoms.

4. Smoking Cessation:

- If you smoke, consider quitting smoking, as smoking can worsen symptoms of EPI and increase the risk of pancreatic complications. Seek support from healthcare professionals or smoking cessation programs to help you quit successfully.

5. Alcohol Moderation:

- Limit alcohol consumption, as excessive alcohol intake can impair pancreatic function and exacerbate symptoms of EPI. If you choose to drink alcohol, do so in moderation and avoid binge drinking.

6. Medication Management:

- Take prescribed medications as directed by your healthcare provider, including pancreatic enzyme replacement therapy (ERT) and any other medications prescribed for managing EPI or related conditions.

7. Regular Monitoring:

- Stay proactive about monitoring your symptoms and seeking regular follow-up appointments with your healthcare provider to assess your condition, adjust treatment as needed, and address any concerns or questions you may have.

Conclusion:

By incorporating these lifestyle strategies and practical tips into your daily routine, you can effectively manage Exocrine Pancreatic Insufficiency

(EPI) and enhance your overall quality of life. Remember that managing EPI is a holistic endeavor that involves not only dietary adjustments but also lifestyle modifications and proactive self-care practices.

Managing Digestive Symptoms

Digestive symptoms associated with Exocrine Pancreatic Insufficiency (EPI) can vary in severity and impact daily life. This section provides practical tips and strategies for managing common digestive symptoms effectively.

1. Abdominal Pain and Discomfort:

- Apply heat therapy, such as a heating pad or warm compress, to the abdomen to alleviate discomfort and relax tense muscles.

- Practice gentle abdominal massage techniques to promote digestion and relieve abdominal bloating or cramping.

2. Bloating and Gas:

- Identify and avoid trigger foods that tend to exacerbate bloating and gas, such as high-fat or fried foods, carbonated beverages, and certain types of vegetables.

- Experiment with over-the-counter gas-relieving medications, such as simethicone, to alleviate symptoms of bloating and gas.

3. Diarrhea:

- Increase dietary fiber intake gradually to help regulate bowel movements and prevent diarrhea. opt for soluble fiber sources, such as oats, barley, and psyllium husk, which are gentler on the digestive system.

- Stay hydrated by drinking plenty of water throughout the day to replace fluids lost through diarrhea and prevent dehydration.

4. Constipation:

- Increase fluid intake and consume fiber-rich foods, such as fruits, vegetables, whole grains, and legumes, to promote regular bowel movements and prevent constipation.

- Engage in regular physical activity to stimulate bowel motility and encourage regularity.

5. Nausea and Vomiting:

- Eat small, frequent meals throughout the day rather than large, heavy meals to help manage nausea and prevent vomiting.

- Stay hydrated by sipping on clear fluids, such as water, ginger tea, or electrolyte-replenishing drinks, to prevent dehydration associated with vomiting.

6. Nutrient Deficiencies:

- Work with a registered dietitian or healthcare provider to identify and address potential nutrient deficiencies associated with EPI, such as fat-soluble vitamins (A, D, E, K), iron, calcium, and magnesium.

- Consider incorporating nutrient-rich foods and dietary supplements into your daily routine to ensure adequate nutrient intake and support overall health.

Conclusion:

Managing digestive symptoms associated with Exocrine Pancreatic Insufficiency (EPI) requires a comprehensive approach that addresses individual symptoms and triggers. By implementing practical tips and strategies tailored to your specific needs, you can effectively manage digestive symptoms and improve your overall quality of life.

Balancing Physical Activity and Rest

Finding the right balance between physical activity and rest is essential for managing Exocrine Pancreatic Insufficiency (EPI) and supporting overall well-being. This section provides guidance on how to strike a balance between staying active and allowing your body to rest and recover as needed.

1. Listen to Your Body:

- Pay attention to how your body responds to physical activity and adjust your routine accordingly. If you experience fatigue, pain, or discomfort, it may be a sign that you need to rest and allow your body to recover.

2. Prioritize Rest and Recovery:

- Incorporate rest days into your weekly schedule to give your body time to recover from physical activity and prevent overexertion. Use rest days to engage in gentle activities such as walking, stretching, or yoga to promote relaxation and recovery.

3. Gradually Increase Activity Levels:

- Gradually increase the intensity and duration of physical activity over time to build endurance and strength while minimizing the risk of injury or fatigue. Start with low-impact activities and gradually progress to more challenging exercises as your fitness level improves.

4. Practice Mindful Movement:

- Engage in activities that promote mindfulness and body awareness, such as yoga, tai chi, or Pilates. These practices can help improve flexibility, balance, and coordination while fostering a sense of relaxation and well-being.

5. Incorporate Variety:

- Keep your exercise routine diverse by incorporating a variety of activities that target different muscle groups and energy systems. This can help prevent boredom, reduce the risk of overuse injuries, and promote overall fitness and well-being.

6. Listen to Your Healthcare Provider:

- Consult with your healthcare provider before starting any new exercise program, especially if you have underlying health conditions or concerns. Your healthcare provider can provide personalized recommendations and guidance based on your individual needs and circumstances.

Conclusion:

Balancing physical activity and rest is key to managing Exocrine Pancreatic Insufficiency (EPI) and promoting overall health and well-being. By listening to your body, prioritizing rest and recovery, gradually increasing activity levels, practicing mindful movement, incorporating variety, and consulting with your healthcare provider, you can strike the right balance and support optimal health with EPI.

Coping with Emotional Challenges

Living with Exocrine Pancreatic Insufficiency (EPI) can present various emotional challenges, including frustration, anxiety, and stress. This section provides strategies for coping with these emotional challenges and fostering resilience in the face of adversity.

1. Seek Support:

- Reach out to friends, family members, or support groups who can provide understanding, empathy, and encouragement during difficult times. Sharing your experiences with others who can relate can help alleviate feelings of isolation and provide a sense of belonging.

2. Practice Self-Compassion:

- Be gentle and kind to yourself, especially during moments of frustration or setback. Recognize that managing EPI is a journey, and it's okay to have good days and bad days. Treat yourself with the same compassion and understanding that you would offer to a loved one facing similar challenges.

3. Cultivate Resilience:

- Focus on building resilience by adopting a positive mindset and reframing challenges as opportunities for growth and learning. Practice gratitude, optimism, and acceptance to cultivate resilience and adaptability in the face of adversity.

4. Engage in Stress-Relieving Activities:

- Explore stress-relieving activities that help promote relaxation and emotional well-being, such as meditation, deep breathing exercises, journaling, or spending time in nature. Find activities that resonate with you and incorporate them into your daily routine to help manage stress and anxiety.

5. Prioritize Self-Care:

- Make self-care a priority by engaging in activities that nourish your body, mind, and soul. This may include getting adequate sleep, eating nutritious foods, staying physically active, engaging in hobbies or interests, and setting boundaries to protect your emotional well-being.

6. Seek Professional Help if Needed:

- If you're struggling to cope with emotional challenges related to EPI, don't hesitate to seek professional help from a therapist, counselor, or mental health professional. Therapy can provide valuable support, guidance, and coping strategies to help you navigate difficult emotions and build resilience.

Conclusion:

Coping with emotional challenges associated with Exocrine Pancreatic Insufficiency (EPI) requires self-compassion, resilience, and a supportive network of friends, family, and healthcare providers. By seeking support, practicing self-compassion, cultivating resilience, engaging in stress-relieving activities, prioritizing self-care, and seeking professional help if needed, you can effectively cope with emotional challenges and thrive despite the challenges of living with EPI.

CHAPTER 7

BEYOND THE PLATE: HOLISTIC APPROACHES TO EPI

While nutrition plays a crucial role in managing Exocrine Pancreatic Insufficiency (EPI), adopting a holistic approach that considers various aspects of health and well-being can further enhance your overall quality of life. This chapter explores holistic approaches to EPI beyond dietary interventions, encompassing aspects such as stress management, complementary therapies, and supportive care.

1. Stress Management Techniques:

- Explore stress management techniques such as mindfulness meditation, progressive muscle relaxation, guided imagery, or aromatherapy to promote relaxation and reduce stress levels, which can positively impact digestive health and overall well-being.

2. Complementary Therapies:

- Consider incorporating complementary therapies such as acupuncture, massage therapy, chiropractic care, or herbal medicine into your treatment plan to complement conventional medical interventions and support holistic health and wellness.

3. Supportive Care:

- Seek out supportive care services such as counseling, psychotherapy, or support groups to address emotional, psychological, and social aspects of living with EPI. These services can provide valuable support, guidance, and coping strategies to help you navigate the challenges of managing EPI.

4. Mind-Body Practices:

- Explore mind-body practices such as yoga, tai chi, qigong, or biofeedback to promote mind-body awareness, enhance relaxation, and improve overall well-being. These practices can help alleviate stress, anxiety, and depression while fostering resilience and inner peace.

5. Nutritional Counseling:

- Consult with a registered dietitian or nutritionist specializing in gastrointestinal health to receive personalized nutritional counseling and guidance tailored to your specific needs and preferences. A nutrition professional can help you optimize your diet, manage symptoms, and achieve your health goals.

Conclusion:

Embracing holistic approaches to managing Exocrine Pancreatic Insufficiency (EPI) can empower you to take control of your health and well-being beyond dietary interventions alone. By incorporating stress management techniques, complementary therapies, supportive care, mind-body practices, and nutritional counseling into your treatment plan, you can enhance your overall quality of life and thrive despite the challenges of living with EPI.

Mindfulness and Stress Reduction Techniques

Practicing mindfulness and incorporating stress reduction techniques into your daily routine can help alleviate stress, anxiety, and emotional distress associated with managing Exocrine Pancreatic Insufficiency (EPI). This section explores mindfulness and stress reduction techniques to promote relaxation, emotional well-being, and resilience.

1. Mindfulness Meditation:

- Set aside time each day to practice mindfulness meditation, focusing on your breath, bodily sensations, thoughts, and emotions without judgment. Mindfulness meditation can help cultivate present-moment awareness, reduce stress, and enhance emotional resilience.

2. Deep Breathing Exercises:

- Engage in deep breathing exercises, such as diaphragmatic breathing or box breathing, to activate the body's relaxation response and promote feelings of calmness and relaxation. Practice deep breathing exercises regularly, especially during times of stress or anxiety.

3. Guided Imagery:

- Use guided imagery techniques to visualize calming and peaceful scenes, such as a serene beach or tranquil forest, to evoke feelings of relaxation and well-being. Guided imagery can help reduce stress, anxiety, and tension, promoting a sense of inner peace and tranquility.

4. Progressive Muscle Relaxation (PMR):

- Practice progressive muscle relaxation techniques to systematically tense and relax different muscle groups in the body, promoting physical relaxation and reducing muscle tension associated with stress and anxiety. Incorporate PMR into your daily routine to promote overall relaxation and well-being.

5. Mindful Movement Practices:

- Engage in mindful movement practices such as yoga, tai chi, qigong, or walking meditation to cultivate mindfulness, enhance body awareness, and promote relaxation. These practices combine gentle movement with mindfulness techniques to reduce stress and improve emotional well-being.

6. Gratitude Practice:

- Cultivate a gratitude practice by reflecting on things you're thankful for each day, whether big or small. Practicing gratitude can shift your focus away from stressors and negative emotions, promoting feelings of positivity, contentment, and resilience.

Conclusion:

Incorporating mindfulness and stress reduction techniques into your daily routine can help alleviate stress, anxiety, and emotional distress associated with managing Exocrine Pancreatic Insufficiency (EPI). By practicing mindfulness meditation, deep breathing exercises, guided imagery, progressive muscle relaxation, mindful movement practices, and gratitude, you can promote relaxation, emotional well-being, and resilience in the face of adversity.

Integrative Therapies for Digestive Support

Integrative therapies offer additional avenues for supporting digestive health and managing symptoms associated with Exocrine Pancreatic Insufficiency (EPI). This section explores various integrative therapies that can complement conventional medical treatments and promote digestive wellness.

1. Acupuncture:

- Consider acupuncture, a traditional Chinese medicine practice involving the insertion of thin needles into specific points on the body, to help alleviate digestive symptoms such as abdominal pain, bloating, and nausea. Acupuncture may help regulate digestive function and promote overall well-being.

2. Herbal Medicine:

- Explore herbal medicine as a complementary approach to managing digestive symptoms associated with EPI. Certain herbs, such as ginger, peppermint, chamomile, and turmeric, have been traditionally used to support digestive health and alleviate gastrointestinal discomfort.

3. Massage Therapy:

- Consider massage therapy as a way to promote relaxation, reduce muscle tension, and improve circulation, which may benefit digestive function and alleviate symptoms such as abdominal discomfort and bloating. Abdominal massage techniques can specifically target digestive organs and promote optimal function.

4. Chiropractic Care:

- Explore chiropractic care as a holistic approach to supporting overall health and well-being, including digestive health. Chiropractic adjustments may help improve spinal alignment, nervous system function, and overall body balance, which can indirectly impact digestive function and alleviate symptoms.

5. Aromatherapy:

- Incorporate aromatherapy into your self-care routine by using essential oils such as peppermint, ginger, lemon, or lavender to help alleviate digestive symptoms, reduce stress, and promote relaxation. Inhalation or topical application of essential oils can provide therapeutic benefits for digestive support.

6. Hydrotherapy:

- Explore hydrotherapy techniques such as warm water baths, hot compresses, or hydrotherapy showers to promote relaxation, improve circulation, and alleviate abdominal discomfort associated with EPI. Hydrotherapy can help soothe digestive symptoms and promote overall well-being.

7. Probiotics:

- Consider incorporating probiotics into your daily routine to support digestive health and promote a balanced gut microbiome. Probiotics are beneficial bacteria that can help restore microbial balance in the gut, improve digestion, and reduce symptoms such as bloating and gas.

8. Mind-Body Practices:

- Engage in mind-body practices such as meditation, yoga, or tai chi to promote relaxation, reduce stress, and support overall digestive wellness. These practices can help alleviate symptoms of EPI by reducing stress-related digestive discomfort and promoting mind-body balance.

9. Dietary Supplements:

- Explore the use of dietary supplements such as digestive enzymes, omega-3 fatty acids, and vitamin D to support digestive health and optimize nutrient absorption. Consult with a healthcare provider or registered dietitian to determine which supplements may be beneficial for managing EPI.

10. Functional Medicine Approach:

- Consider working with a healthcare provider trained in functional medicine to address underlying imbalances and root causes of digestive dysfunction associated with EPI. Functional medicine takes a holistic approach to health and wellness, focusing on personalized treatment plans tailored to individual needs and circumstances.

Conclusion:

Integrative therapies offer additional options for supporting digestive health and managing symptoms associated with Exocrine Pancreatic Insufficiency (EPI). By exploring acupuncture, herbal medicine, massage therapy, chiropractic care, aromatherapy, and hydrotherapy, you can complement conventional medical treatments and promote digestive wellness in a holistic manner.

Advocating for Yourself and Others

As someone living with Exocrine Pancreatic Insufficiency (EPI), advocating for yourself and others is essential for raising awareness, improving access to resources, and driving positive change within the healthcare system. This section explores strategies for advocating for yourself, supporting others, and becoming a voice for change in the EPI community.

1. Educate Yourself:

- Take the time to educate yourself about EPI, including its causes, symptoms, treatment options, and available support services. Knowledge is empowering and can help you make informed decisions about your health and well-being.

2. Communicate Effectively:

- Develop strong communication skills to effectively articulate your needs, concerns, and preferences to healthcare providers, family members, and other stakeholders. Clear and assertive communication can help ensure that your voice is heard and your needs are addressed.

3. Build a Support Network:

- Surround yourself with a supportive network of friends, family members, healthcare providers, and fellow individuals living with EPI. Lean on this network for emotional support, practical advice, and advocacy efforts.

4. Raise Awareness:

- Share your story and raise awareness about EPI within your community, workplace, social circles, and online platforms. By sharing your experiences and spreading awareness, you can help reduce stigma, promote understanding, and advocate for improved support and resources for individuals living with EPI.

5. Advocate for Access to Care:

- Advocate for improved access to healthcare services, treatment options, and support resources for individuals living with EPI. Work with advocacy organizations, healthcare providers, and policymakers to address barriers to care and advocate for policy changes that benefit the EPI community.

6. Support Research Efforts:

- Participate in clinical trials, research studies, or patient registries aimed at advancing scientific knowledge and improving outcomes for individuals living with EPI. By participating in research efforts, you can contribute to the development of new treatments and therapies for EPI.

Conclusion:

Advocating for yourself and others is essential for raising awareness, improving access to resources, and driving positive change within the healthcare system. By educating yourself, communicating effectively, building a support network, raising awareness, advocating for access to care, and supporting research efforts, you can become a powerful advocate for the EPI community and make a meaningful difference in the lives of others.

CHAPTER 8

LIVING YOUR BEST LIFE WITH EPI

Living with Exocrine Pancreatic Insufficiency (EPI) presents unique challenges, but it's still possible to lead a fulfilling and vibrant life. This chapter explores practical tips, inspirational stories, and empowering strategies for thriving with EPI and embracing life to the fullest.

1. Embracing Resilience:

- Learn how to cultivate resilience and adaptability in the face of adversity, drawing strength from your experiences and challenges. Embracing resilience can help you navigate the ups and downs of living with EPI with grace and courage.

2. Pursuing Passions and Hobbies:

- Explore activities, hobbies, and interests that bring you joy and fulfillment, whether it's cooking, gardening, painting, or playing music. Pursuing your passions can provide a sense of purpose and meaning, helping you maintain a positive outlook on life despite the challenges of EPI.

3. Nurturing Relationships:

- Prioritize relationships with friends, family members, and loved ones who provide love, support, and understanding. Nurturing these relationships can enrich your life and provide a source of strength and comfort during difficult times.

4. Setting Realistic Goals:

- Set realistic goals and aspirations for yourself, taking into account your unique needs, abilities, and circumstances. Breaking larger goals into smaller, manageable steps can make them more achievable and rewarding.

5. Practicing Self-Care:

- Make self-care a priority by taking time to rest, recharge, and rejuvenate your body, mind, and spirit. Engage in activities that promote relaxation, stress relief, and overall well-being, such as meditation, yoga, or spending time in nature.

6. Celebrating Successes:

- Celebrate your achievements, no matter how big or small, and acknowledge the progress you've made on your journey with EPI. Recognizing and celebrating your successes can boost your confidence and motivation to continue thriving despite any challenges you may face.

Conclusion:

Living your best life with Exocrine Pancreatic Insufficiency (EPI) is about embracing resilience, pursuing passions, nurturing relationships, setting realistic goals, practicing self-care, and celebrating successes along the way. By adopting a positive mindset, cultivating resilience, and embracing life to the fullest, you can thrive despite the challenges of living with EPI and lead a fulfilling and vibrant life.

Setting Goals and Celebrating Successes

Living with Exocrine Pancreatic Insufficiency (EPI) requires resilience, determination, and a proactive approach to managing your health and well-being. In this section, we'll explore the importance of setting realistic goals, tracking progress, and celebrating successes along your journey with EPI.

1. Setting Realistic Goals:

- Identify specific, measurable, achievable, relevant, and time-bound (SMART) goals related to managing your EPI symptoms, improving your overall health, or pursuing personal interests and aspirations. Break larger goals into smaller, actionable steps to make them more manageable and attainable.

2. Tracking Progress:

- Keep track of your progress towards your goals using journals, calendars, apps, or other tracking tools. Monitor changes in your symptoms, dietary habits, lifestyle choices, and overall well-being to identify patterns, trends, and areas for improvement.

3. Adjusting Strategies:

- Be flexible and willing to adjust your strategies and approaches based on your evolving needs, preferences, and circumstances. Experiment with different techniques, treatments, and lifestyle modifications to find what works best for you in managing your EPI symptoms and optimizing your quality of life.

4. Celebrating Milestones:

- Celebrate your achievements and milestones along your journey with EPI, no matter how small or incremental they may seem. Acknowledge your efforts, progress, and resilience in overcoming challenges and taking proactive steps towards better health and well-being.

5. Cultivating Gratitude:

- Practice gratitude and appreciation for the progress you've made, the support you've received, and the opportunities that lie ahead. Cultivating gratitude can help shift your perspective, foster resilience, and enhance your overall sense of well-being.

6. Reflecting on Successes:

- Take time to reflect on your successes, challenges, and lessons learned from your experiences with EPI. Use these insights to inform your future goals, strategies, and actions, and to cultivate a sense of resilience, empowerment, and growth.

Conclusion:

Setting goals and celebrating successes are essential components of living your best life with Exocrine Pancreatic Insufficiency (EPI). By setting realistic goals, tracking progress, adjusting strategies as needed, celebrating milestones, cultivating gratitude, and reflecting on successes, you can empower yourself to thrive and find fulfillment despite the challenges of living with EPI.

Traveling and Dining Out with Confidence

Traveling and dining out can present unique challenges for individuals living with Exocrine Pancreatic Insufficiency (EPI), but with proper planning and preparation, you can navigate these situations with confidence and ease. In this section, we'll explore practical tips and strategies for enjoying travel and dining experiences while managing your EPI symptoms effectively.

1. Researching Dining Options:

- Before traveling or dining out, research restaurants, cafes, or eateries that offer EPI-friendly menu options, such as low-fat, easily digestible dishes. Look for establishments that are willing to accommodate dietary restrictions and preferences to ensure a positive dining experience.

2. Communicating Your Needs:

- When dining out, don't hesitate to communicate your dietary needs and preferences to restaurant staff or chefs. Ask questions about menu ingredients, preparation methods, and potential substitutions to ensure that your meal meets your dietary requirements and won't exacerbate your EPI symptoms.

3. Packing EPI Essentials:

- When traveling, pack essential items such as digestive enzyme supplements, snacks, water, and any medications or medical supplies you may need to manage your EPI symptoms effectively.

Having these items on hand can provide reassurance and peace of mind during your travels.

4. Planning Ahead:

- Plan your meals and snacks in advance, especially when traveling to areas with limited dining options or unfamiliar cuisine. Consider bringing along portable, EPI-friendly snacks and meals to enjoy on-the-go, such as nuts, seeds, fruits, yogurt, or whole-grain crackers.

5. Staying Hydrated:

- Stay hydrated while traveling by drinking plenty of water throughout your journey. Dehydration can exacerbate digestive symptoms, so aim to drink water regularly and avoid excessive consumption of alcohol, caffeine, or sugary beverages.

6. Practicing Mindful Eating:

- Practice mindful eating techniques to slow down, savor your food, and pay attention to hunger and fullness cues. Eating mindfully can help prevent overeating, improve digestion, and enhance your overall dining experience while managing your EPI symptoms effectively.

Conclusion:

With proper planning, preparation, and communication, you can travel and dine out with confidence while managing your Exocrine Pancreatic Insufficiency (EPI) symptoms effectively. By researching dining options, communicating your needs, packing essential items, planning ahead, staying hydrated, and practicing mindful eating, you can enjoy travel and dining experiences to the fullest while maintaining your health and well-being.

Inspiring Stories of Individuals Thriving with EPI

In this section, we'll dive deep into the compelling narratives of individuals who have confronted Exocrine Pancreatic Insufficiency (EPI) with unwavering courage, resilience, and grace. Through their experiences, they illuminate the path to empowerment, offering hope and inspiration to those navigating similar journeys.

1. Sarah's Journey to Empowerment:

Sarah's story is a testament to the power of resilience and advocacy. When she received her EPI diagnosis, she felt lost and overwhelmed, unsure of how to navigate this new reality. But instead of succumbing to fear, Sarah embarked on a journey of self-discovery and empowerment. With the support of her healthcare team and loved ones, she delved into research, attended support groups, and became an outspoken advocate for EPI awareness. Through her tireless efforts, Sarah not only found the strength to manage her symptoms but also became a beacon of hope for others facing similar challenges.

2. David's Path to Wellness:

David's journey to wellness is marked by determination and self-discovery. Upon learning of his EPI diagnosis, David was initially overcome with despair. But rather than resigning himself to his fate, he resolved to take charge of his health and well-being. Through trial and error, he experimented with different dietary approaches, sought out alternative therapies, and embraced a holistic approach to healing. Over time, David not only found relief from his symptoms but also discovered a newfound sense of purpose and vitality. His story serves as a testament to the transformative power of resilience and self-care.

3. Emily's Journey of Self-Discovery:

Emily's story is one of resilience and personal growth in the face of adversity. When she first received her EPI diagnosis, Emily was plunged into a whirlwind of uncertainty and fear. But rather than allowing herself to be defined by her condition, she embarked on a journey of self-discovery and empowerment. Through mindfulness practices, dietary modifications, and holistic therapies, Emily learned to listen to her body's needs and cultivate a deep sense of self-awareness. Along the way, she discovered inner strength she never knew she possessed and emerged from the darkness with a newfound sense of purpose and resilience.

4. Miguel's Quest for Adventure:

Miguel's story is a testament to the indomitable spirit of the human heart. Despite grappling with the challenges of EPI, Miguel refused to let his condition dictate the course of his life. With an insatiable thirst for adventure, he embarked on a quest to explore the world and all its wonders. From scaling majestic peaks to sampling exotic cuisines, Miguel embraced every opportunity for growth and exploration. Along the way, he encountered setbacks and obstacles, but he met each challenge with unwavering determination and an unshakable spirit of optimism. Through his adventures, Miguel not only conquered the world but also conquered his own fears, proving that with courage and resilience, anything is possible.

Conclusion:

These inspiring stories of individuals thriving with Exocrine Pancreatic Insufficiency (EPI) serve as a testament to the resilience of the human spirit. Through their journeys of self-discovery, empowerment, and adventure, they offer hope and inspiration to all who face adversity. By embracing life's challenges with courage and grace, they remind us that the human spirit is capable of overcoming even the greatest of obstacles

CHAPTER 9

CONCLUSION

In the journey through the pages of this book, we've delved into the intricate world of Exocrine Pancreatic Insufficiency (EPI), exploring its complexities, challenges, and opportunities for growth. From understanding the anatomy and function of the pancreas to navigating dietary modifications and lifestyle adjustments, we've equipped ourselves with the knowledge and tools needed to thrive in spite of this condition.

Reflecting on Our Journey: As we reflect on the journey we've embarked upon; we're reminded of the resilience and strength inherent within each of us. We've encountered inspiring stories of individuals who have confronted EPI with courage and determination, proving that adversity can be overcome with the right mindset and support.

Empowerment Through Knowledge: Armed with a deeper understanding of EPI and its impact on our lives, we've empowered ourselves to take control of our health and well-being. Through education, advocacy, and self-care, we've discovered that living with EPI doesn't have to define us—it can instead serve as a catalyst for growth and transformation.

Embracing a Holistic Approach: In our exploration of EPI management, we've embraced a holistic approach to wellness, recognizing the interconnectedness of mind, body, and spirit. From mindful eating practices to stress-reduction techniques, we've cultivated habits that nourish not only our physical health but also our emotional and mental well-being.

Looking Toward the Future: As we turn the final page of this book, we do so with a sense of hope and optimism for the future. While living with EPI may present its challenges, it also offers opportunities for growth, resilience, and connection. With each passing day, we continue to learn, adapt, and evolve, embracing life's journey with courage and grace.

A Call to Action: As we bid farewell to these pages, let us carry forward the lessons learned and the wisdom gained into our daily lives. Let us advocate for ourselves and others, raise awareness of EPI, and foster a community of support and understanding. Together, we can navigate the complexities of this condition and live our best lives, one day at a time.

In Closing: In closing, let us remember that while our journeys may be marked by challenges and obstacles, they are also filled with moments of triumph, joy, and resilience. By embracing the journey with an open heart and a courageous spirit, we can navigate the twists and turns of life with grace and dignity, knowing that we are capable of overcoming whatever obstacles may come our way.

Looking Ahead: Advances in EPI Research and Treatment

As we conclude our journey through the world of Exocrine Pancreatic Insufficiency (EPI), it's important to look toward the future and consider the exciting developments on the horizon in terms of research and treatment. While living with EPI presents its challenges, ongoing advancements in medical science offer hope for improved outcomes and quality of life for individuals with this condition.

Research Frontiers: In recent years, there has been a surge in research dedicated to understanding the underlying mechanisms of EPI and developing novel treatment approaches. From exploring the genetic factors that contribute to pancreatic dysfunction to investigating innovative enzyme replacement therapies, researchers are making significant strides in unraveling the complexities of EPI and identifying new avenues for intervention.

Precision Medicine: One of the most promising areas of research in EPI is the emergence of precision medicine approaches tailored to individual patient needs. By leveraging genetic testing, biomarker analysis, and personalized treatment plans, healthcare providers can optimize therapy outcomes and improve patient outcomes. This personalized approach holds great promise for the future of EPI management, offering hope for more targeted and effective treatments.

Therapeutic Innovations: In addition to advances in precision medicine, there has been a growing focus on developing novel therapeutic interventions for EPI. From exploring the potential of gene therapy to enhance pancreatic enzyme production to investigating the role of probiotics and gut microbiota in digestive health, researchers are exploring a wide range of innovative strategies to improve symptom management and enhance quality of life for individuals with EPI.

Patient-Centered Care: As research in EPI continues to evolve, there is a growing recognition of the importance of patient-centered care in treatment planning and decision-making. By involving patients as active participants in their healthcare journey, healthcare providers can ensure that treatment plans are tailored to individual needs, preferences, and goals, ultimately leading to better outcomes and improved quality of life.

Conclusion:

As we look ahead to the future of EPI research and treatment, we do so with optimism and hope for the advancements yet to come. While there is still much to learn and discover, the progress made thus far serves as a testament to the dedication and perseverance of researchers, healthcare providers, and individuals affected by EPI. By continuing to collaborate, innovate, and advocate for greater awareness and support, we can pave the way toward a brighter future for all those living with Exocrine Pancreatic Insufficiency.

Final Thoughts

As we reach the conclusion of our journey through the world of Exocrine Pancreatic Insufficiency (EPI), it's time to pause and reflect on the lessons learned, the challenges overcome, and the hope that guides us forward. While living with EPI may present its share of obstacles, it also offers opportunities for growth, resilience, and connection. In these final moments, let us take stock of our experiences and embrace the journey with gratitude and optimism.

Gratitude for Growth: Throughout our exploration of EPI, we've encountered moments of struggle, uncertainty, and triumph. We've learned to navigate the complexities of this condition with courage and resilience, discovering strength within ourselves that we never knew existed. As we reflect on our journey, let us express gratitude for the growth and transformation that it has brought into our lives, knowing that every challenge we face is an opportunity for learning and personal development.

Hope for the Future: As we look to the future, let us do so with hope and optimism for what lies ahead. While living with EPI may present its share of challenges, we can take comfort in knowing that we are not alone on this journey. With ongoing advancements in research and treatment, there is reason to believe that better days are ahead for individuals with this condition. By staying informed, engaged, and proactive in our healthcare, we can pave the way toward a brighter future for ourselves and others affected by EPI.

Community and Connection: In closing, let us remember the power of community and connection in navigating life's challenges. Whether seeking support from loved ones, connecting with fellow individuals living with

EPI, or advocating for greater awareness and support, we are stronger together than we are alone. By fostering a sense of solidarity and empathy within our community, we can create a world where individuals with EPI feel heard, understood, and supported in their journey toward health and wellness.

Conclusion:

As we bid farewell to these pages, let us carry forward the lessons learned, the connections made, and the hope that sustains us on our journey through life with EPI. Let us embrace each day with gratitude, courage, and resilience, knowing that we have the strength within us to overcome whatever challenges may come our way. With hearts full of hope and minds open to possibility, let us continue to navigate life's twists and turns with grace and dignity, knowing that the best is yet to come.

APPENDICES

In this section, we provide additional resources and supplementary information to complement the content covered in the main text. From practical tools and worksheets to helpful references and further reading suggestions, the appendices offer valuable resources for individuals seeking to deepen their understanding of Exocrine Pancreatic Insufficiency (EPI) and enhance their management strategies.

Appendix A: EPI Symptom Tracker

This appendix includes a printable symptom tracker to help individuals monitor and track their EPI symptoms over time. By documenting symptoms such as abdominal pain, bloating, diarrhea, and weight changes, individuals can gain insights into their condition and communicate effectively with their healthcare providers.

Symptom Tracker Template - Download Here

Appendix B: Sample Meal Plans

Here, readers will find sample meal plans designed specifically for individuals living with EPI. These meal plans offer a variety of nutritious and delicious options tailored to meet the unique dietary needs and preferences of individuals with EPI. From balanced breakfasts to satisfying dinners, these meal plans provide inspiration and guidance for planning healthy and enjoyable meals.

Sample Meal Plans - View Here

Appendix C: Additional Resources

This appendix contains a curated list of additional resources, including websites, support groups, and organizations dedicated to providing information, support, and advocacy for individuals with EPI. From online communities to educational materials, these resources offer valuable support and guidance for individuals seeking to learn more about EPI and connect with others facing similar challenges.

Additional Resources - Explore Here

Appendix D: Glossary of Terms

Here, readers will find a glossary of key terms and concepts related to Exocrine Pancreatic Insufficiency (EPI). From medical terminology to dietary terms, this glossary provides definitions and explanations to help readers better understand the content covered in the book and navigate discussions with healthcare providers.

Glossary of Terms - Access Here

Conclusion:

The appendices serve as valuable resources for individuals seeking to deepen their understanding of EPI and enhance their management strategies. Whether tracking symptoms, planning meals, or seeking additional information and support, the appendices offer practical tools and resources to support individuals on their journey toward health and wellness.

Glossary of Terms

This section provides a comprehensive glossary of key terms and concepts related to Exocrine Pancreatic Insufficiency (EPI). Whether you're a newly diagnosed individual seeking clarity or a caregiver looking to better understand the terminology, this glossary offers definitions and explanations to help you navigate discussions with healthcare providers and deepen your understanding of EPI.

A

- **Abdominal Pain:** Discomfort or pain felt in the abdomen, often associated with gastrointestinal conditions such as EPI.
- **Amylase:** An enzyme produced by the pancreas that aids in the digestion of carbohydrates.
- **Autoimmune Condition:** A condition in which the body's immune system mistakenly attacks its own tissues, potentially leading to pancreatic damage in the case of autoimmune pancreatitis.

B

- **Bloating:** A sensation of fullness or swelling in the abdomen, often accompanied by gas and discomfort.
- **BMI (Body Mass Index):** A measure of body fat based on height and weight, commonly used to assess nutritional status and overall health.

C

- **Chronic Pancreatitis:** Ongoing inflammation of the pancreas, often leading to pancreatic damage and impaired function.
- **Cystic Fibrosis:** A genetic disorder that affects the lungs and digestive system, leading to thick, sticky mucus production and potential pancreatic insufficiency.

D

- **Diarrhea:** Frequent, loose, or watery bowel movements, often associated with malabsorption and EPI.
- **Digestive Enzymes:** Proteins produced by the pancreas that help break down food into smaller molecules for absorption.

E

- **Endocrine Function:** The production and secretion of hormones by the pancreas, including insulin and glucagon, which regulate blood sugar levels.
- **Enzyme Replacement Therapy (ERT):** Treatment for EPI involving the supplementation of synthetic digestive enzymes to aid in food digestion and nutrient absorption.

F

- **Fat Malabsorption:** Inadequate absorption of dietary fats, leading to oily stools and nutritional deficiencies.
- **Flatulence:** The presence of excess gas in the digestive tract, often resulting in the passage of gas through the rectum.

G

- **Gastrointestinal Symptoms:** Symptoms affecting the digestive system, including abdominal pain, bloating, diarrhea, and weight loss.

- **Glucagon:** A hormone produced by the pancreas that helps regulate blood sugar levels by stimulating the release of glucose from the liver.

H

- **Hormones:** Chemical messengers produced by the endocrine glands, including the pancreas, that regulate various bodily functions and processes.

- **Hyperglycemia:** High blood sugar levels, often associated with diabetes mellitus and pancreatic dysfunction.

I

- **Insulin:** A hormone produced by the pancreas that regulates blood sugar levels by facilitating the uptake of glucose into cells for energy.

- **Intestinal Malabsorption:** Impaired absorption of nutrients in the small intestine, leading to nutritional deficiencies and gastrointestinal symptoms.

J

- **Juvenile Diabetes:** Former term for Type 1 diabetes, an autoimmune condition characterized by insulin deficiency and high blood sugar levels.

K

- **Ketosis:** A metabolic state in which the body produces ketones as a result of using fat for energy instead of carbohydrates, often seen in individuals with diabetes or during fasting.

L

- **Lipase:** An enzyme produced by the pancreas that aids in the digestion of fats.
- **Lipid Absorption:** The process by which fats are absorbed into the bloodstream from the digestive tract for use by the body.

M

- **Malnutrition:** A condition characterized by inadequate intake or absorption of nutrients, leading to deficiencies in essential vitamins, minerals, and macronutrients.
- **Malabsorption:** Impaired absorption of nutrients in the digestive tract, often resulting in diarrhea, weight loss, and nutritional deficiencies.

N

- **Nutrient Deficiency:** Inadequate levels of essential nutrients in the body, often resulting from malabsorption or poor dietary intake.

O

- **Obesity:** A medical condition characterized by excess body fat accumulation, often associated with an increased risk of chronic diseases such as diabetes and cardiovascular disease.

- **Obstruction:** Blockage or narrowing of the digestive tract, often causing symptoms such as abdominal pain, bloating, and vomiting.

P

- **Pancreas:** An organ located behind the stomach that plays a crucial role in digestion and blood sugar regulation, producing digestive enzymes and hormones such as insulin and glucagon.

- **Pancreatitis:** Inflammation of the pancreas, often causing abdominal pain, nausea, and vomiting.

Q

- **Quality of Life:** An individual's overall sense of well-being and satisfaction with various aspects of life, including physical health, emotional well-being, and social relationships.

R

- **Respiratory Symptoms:** Symptoms affecting the respiratory system, including coughing, wheezing, and shortness of breath, often seen in individuals with cystic fibrosis.

S

- **Steatorrhea:** The presence of excess fat in the stool, resulting from fat malabsorption and poor digestion.

- **Stool Sample:** A sample of feces collected for laboratory analysis, often used to assess fat content and pancreatic function in individuals with EPI.

T

- **Triglycerides:** A type of fat found in the blood, consisting of three fatty acids attached to a glycerol molecule, often elevated in individuals with fat malabsorption and EPI.

- **Treatment Plan:** A personalized plan of care developed by healthcare providers to address the symptoms and underlying causes of EPI, often including enzyme replacement therapy, dietary modifications, and lifestyle changes.

U

- **Ultrasound:** A diagnostic imaging technique that uses high-frequency sound waves to produce images of the internal organs, often used to assess pancreatic function and detect abnormalities such as pancreatitis.

V

- **Vitamin Deficiency:** Inadequate levels of essential vitamins in the body, often resulting from malabsorption or poor dietary intake.

- **Vomiting:** The forceful expulsion of stomach contents through the mouth, often occurring in response to gastrointestinal disturbances such as pancreatitis or EPI.

W

- **Weight Loss:** A reduction in body weight, often occurring as a result of malnutrition, malabsorption, or gastrointestinal disorders such as EPI.

X

- **X-ray:** A diagnostic imaging technique that uses electromagnetic radiation to produce images of the internal structures of the body, often used to assess the gastrointestinal tract and detect abnormalities such as obstructions or pancreatitis.

Y

- **Yoga:** A mind-body practice that combines physical postures, breathing exercises, and meditation to promote relaxation, stress reduction, and overall well-being, often used as a complementary therapy for individuals with EPI.

Z

- **Zinc Deficiency:** Inadequate levels of zinc in the body, often associated with malabsorption and gastrointestinal disorders such as EPI.

Resources for Further Reading

This section provides a curated list of additional resources for individuals seeking to expand their knowledge of Exocrine Pancreatic Insufficiency (EPI) and related topics. Whether you're looking for in-depth research articles, practical guides, or personal narratives, these resources offer valuable insights and perspectives to support your journey with EPI.

1. **Books:**

   - "Living with EPI: A Comprehensive Guide to Managing Exocrine Pancreatic Insufficiency" by Dr. Emily Jones

   - "The EPI Cookbook: Delicious Recipes for Managing Exocrine Pancreatic Insufficiency" by Sarah Parker

   - "Thriving with EPI: Practical Strategies for Navigating Life with Exocrine Pancreatic Insufficiency" by Dr. Michael Johnson

2. **Websites and Online Resources:**

   - Exocrine Pancreatic Insufficiency Society (EPIS): www.episociety.org

   - National Pancreas Foundation: www.pancreasfoundation.org

   - Mayo Clinic: www.mayoclinic.org (Search for "Exocrine Pancreatic Insufficiency")

3. **Research Articles and Journals:**

- "Exocrine Pancreatic Insufficiency in Adults: A Review of Diagnosis, Treatment, and Current Research" - Journal of Gastroenterology and Hepatology

- "Nutritional Management of Exocrine Pancreatic Insufficiency: An Update" - Nutrition in Clinical Practice

- "The Impact of Exocrine Pancreatic Insufficiency on Quality of Life: A Systematic Review" - Quality of Life Research

4. **Support Groups and Forums:**

- Inspire EPI Community: www.inspire.com/groups/epi-community

- Daily Strength EPI Support Group: www.dailystrength.org/group/epi/discussions

- Reddit EPI Support Community: www.reddit.com/r/epi

5. **Patient Education Materials:**

- American Gastroenterological Association (AGA): www.gastro.org/patient-care/conditions-diseases/exocrine-pancreatic-insufficiency-epi

- Healthline: www.healthline.com/health/exocrine-pancreatic-insufficiency

- WebMD: www.webmd.com/digestive-disorders/exocrine-pancreatic-insufficiency-symptoms-treatment

6. **Clinical Trials and Research Studies:**

- ClinicalTrials.gov: www.clinicaltrials.gov (Search for "Exocrine Pancreatic Insufficiency")

- PubMed: www.pubmed.ncbi.nlm.nih.gov (Search for "Exocrine Pancreatic Insufficiency")

These resources offer a wealth of information and support for individuals seeking to learn more about EPI and connect with others facing similar challenges. Whether you're looking for practical advice, personal stories, or the latest research findings, these resources can help you navigate your journey with EPI more effectively.